Handbook of
NEUROLOGICAL DRUGS

Handbook of
NEUROLOGICAL DRUGS

D Vasudevan
MD(General Medicine) DM(Neurology) FRCP
Professor and Head
Department of Neurology
Saveetha Medical College
Chennai, Tamil Nadu, India

S Vinoth Kanna
MD(General Medicine) DM(Neurology)
Professor
Department of Neurology
Saveetha Medical College
Chennai, Tamil Nadu, India

M Sathish Kumar
MD(General Medicine) DM(Neurology)
Assistant Professor
Department of Neurology
Saveetha Medical College
Chennai, Tamil Nadu, India

M Nirumal Khumar
MD(General Medicine)
DM(Neurology) DrNB(Neurology) FEBN
Assistant Professor
Department of Neurology
Saveetha Medical College
Chennai, Tamil Nadu, India

Forewords

CU Velmurugendran
AV Srinivasan

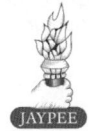

JAYPEE BROTHERS MEDICAL PUBLISHERS
The Health Sciences Publisher
New Delhi | London

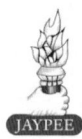

Jaypee Brothers Medical Publishers (P) Ltd

Headquarters
Jaypee Brothers Medical Publishers (P) Ltd
23/23-B, Ansari Road, Daryaganj
New Delhi 110 002, India
Phone: +91-11-23272143, +91-11-23272703
+91-11-23282021, +91-11-23245672
E-mail: jaypee@jaypeebrothers.com

Corporate Office
Jaypee Brothers Medical Publishers (P) Ltd
4838/24, Ansari Road, Daryaganj
New Delhi 110 002, India
Phone: +91-11-43574357
Fax: +91-11-43574314
E-mail: jaypee@jaypeebrothers.com

Overseas Office
JP Medical Ltd
83 Victoria Street, London
SW1H 0HW (UK)
Phone: +44 20 3170 8910
E-mail: info@jpmedpub.com

EU GPSR Authorised Representative
Logos Europe, 9 rue Nicolas Poussin
17000, La Rochelle, France
Phone: +33 (0) 6 67 93 73 78
E-mail: Contact@logoseurope.eu

Website: www.jaypeebrothers.com
Website: www.jaypeedigital.com

© 2025, Jaypee Brothers Medical Publishers

The views and opinions expressed in this book are solely those of the original contributor(s)/author(s) and do not necessarily represent those of editor(s) or publisher of the book.

All rights reserved. No part of this publication may be reproduced, stored or transmitted in any form or by any means, electronic, mechanical, photocopying, recording or otherwise, without the prior permission in writing of the publishers.

All brand names and product names used in this book are trade names, service marks, trademarks or registered trademarks of their respective owners. The publisher is not associated with any product or vendor mentioned in this book.

Medical knowledge and practice change constantly. This book is designed to provide accurate, authoritative information about the subject matter in question. However, readers are advised to check the most current information available on procedures included and check information from the manufacturer of each product to be administered, to verify the recommended dose, formula, method and duration of administration, adverse effects and contraindications. It is the responsibility of the practitioner to take all appropriate safety precautions. Neither the publisher nor the author(s)/editor(s) assume any liability for any injury and/or damage to persons or property arising from or related to use of material in this book.

This book is sold on the understanding that the publisher is not engaged in providing professional medical services. If such advice or services are required, the services of a competent medical professional should be sought.

Every effort has been made where necessary to contact holders of copyright to obtain permission to reproduce copyright material. If any have been inadvertently overlooked, the publisher will be pleased to make the necessary arrangements at the first opportunity.

Inquiries for bulk sales may be solicited at: jaypee@jaypeebrothers.com

Handbook of Neurological Drugs / D Vasudevan, S Vinoth Kanna, M Sathish Kumar, M Nirumal Khumar

First Edition: **2025**

ISBN: 978-93-6616-713-8

Printed in India at Sterling Graphics Pvt. Ltd.

Foreword

Neurology is both a science and an art. It delves deeply into the intricate workings of the nervous system while also requiring a nuanced understanding of the human condition. Hence, the drugs used in neuroscience play a pivotal role in restoring neural identity. It is with immense pleasure that I write the foreword for Professor Vasudevan's groundbreaking textbook *"Handbook of Neurological Drugs."* This meticulously compiled volume is more than just a reference tool. It is an essential guide for clinicians at all stages of their careers.

Professor Vasudevan and his team's work stands out for its thorough and systematic approach. By tabulating drugs used in neurology in an alphabetical order, the textbook provides an unparalleled and never-seen-before level of organization and accessibility. Each entry offers a comprehensive overview of pharmacokinetics, pharmacodynamics, indications, contraindications, dosage, mechanisms of action, and side effects. The authors have done extensive research to compile the details in the book and have presented it in an easy, understandable manner. This meticulous attention to detail ensures that practitioners can swiftly locate critical information and make informed decisions about patient care, on a daily basis.

What makes this textbook truly unique is its dual utility. For seasoned neurologists, it serves as a quick and reliable reference, streamlining the process of drug selection and management. For young neurophysicians and trainees, it offers an invaluable educational resource, facilitating a deeper understanding of drug mechanisms and therapeutic applications. The clarity and structure of the information presented allow for both efficient recall and comprehensive learning.

In a field as dynamic and complex as neurology, where new drugs and treatment protocols are continually evolving, having a resource that combines ease of use with in-depth knowledge is invaluable. Professor Vasudevan's *"Handbook of Neurological Drugs"* is destined to become a cornerstone in the libraries of neurology professionals, providing both practical guidance and educational enrichment.

In conclusion, this textbook reflects not only Professor Vasudevan and his team's expertise but also their dedication to advancing the field of neurology. It is a commendable contribution that will undoubtedly aid countless clinicians in their pursuit of excellence in patient care.

CU Velmurugendran
Padma Shri Awardee
MD(Medicine) DM(Neurology)
PhD DSc(Hon) FAMS FIAN FRCP
Emeritus Professor
The Tamil Nadu Dr. MGR Medical University
Former Head and Professor of Neurology
Institute of Neurology, Madras Medical College
Former Director of Neurology, SRIHER
Chennai, Tamil Nadu, India

Foreword

I am delighted to write this foreword to the first edition of *"Handbook of Neurological Drugs"*. I believe it is the first of its kind in putting the therapeutic armamentarium of neurological medicine within easy reach. It helps the busy practitioner and the student alike. This book has been written with great care and accuracy by the authors, experts in the neurological field, and meticulously backed by evidence-based medicine. It provides easy access to practical information about day-to-day problems in patient care for quick reference to advances in neurotherapeutics. I sincerely appreciate the authors who have done a sterling service in this regard. The aim of providing information about all drugs and biologicals used in neurological practice is indeed a daunting task and I am happy to note that the authors have met this challenge successfully which is evident in the thoughtful arrangement of the book in two sections. Ease of use is a distinct hallmark, the first section being an alphabetical ordering of drugs with precise discussion of each drug, namely its pharmacodynamics, pharmacokinetics, usefulness, dosing, adverse effects and use in special populations and special situations. The second section provides a ready reference of the commonly used neurological medications in disease categories along with their classifications. This is indeed a unique and strong feature of this book. I am pretty sure that this book will definitely increase the scope, versatility, and effectiveness of treatment. I strongly recommend this book to every practitioner, novice, and expert alike and I am confident that it will find a place on the desk of all neurologists as a ready and easy reference for perfection in the management of neurological disorders.

AV Srinivasan
MD(Medicine) DM(Neurology) PhD
FAAN FIAN DSc(Hon) FRCP(London)
Emeritus Professor
The Tamil Nadu Dr MGR Medical University
Former Head and Professor of Neurology
Institute of Neurology, Madras Medical College
Chennai, Tamil Nadu, India

Preface

With the rapid strides made in the recent years in the therapeutic armamentarium of medicine in general and neurology in particular, there has been an explosion in the number of drugs and biologicals available to the practicing neurologist and the trainee to choose from. Although by itself, the availability of numerous options may increase the scope, versatility, and effectiveness of treatment, at times it leaves the practitioner confounded and bewildered.

This book *"Handbook of Neurological Drugs"* aims to categorize these drugs and provide an instant reference for the neurologist. The book is designed in two sections. The first section arranges the drugs and biologicals in an alphabetical order with a brief description of the indications, contraindications, relevant pharmacokinetics, and pharmacodynamics information and special situations and populations. The second section provides a disease- or condition-based categorization of the drugs with appropriate classifications where necessary.

Although by no means comprehensive, our aim in this book is to provide a ready reference of the commonly used neurological medications as well as those used in special situations. We have consciously excluded categories like antihypertensives, statins, antibiotics, antineoplastic drugs, etc., as these are not specifically neurological and the information regarding these drugs is easily available from other sources. Only drugs with robust scientific evidence, which are of use in neurological conditions, are included and certain drugs/preparations, although used popularly, lacking in such evidence have been excluded.

We are deeply grateful to all our teachers for their encouragement and guidance, colleagues, students, and patients from whom we always learn anew. We are thankful to our family members for their constant support. We owe special thanks to Mr Ashish Kumar (Senior Business Development Manager) and Piyush Bhatnagar (Development Editor) of Jaypee Brothers Medical Publishers for pushing and encouraging us to finish this book in time.

D Vasudevan
S Vinoth Kanna
M Sathish Kumar
M Nirumal Khumar

Contents

SECTION 1: Drugs Used in Neurology

A

Acenocoumarol	3
Acetazolamide	4
Acyclovir	4
Aducanumab	5
Albuterol	6
Alemtuzumab	7
Alglucosidase Alfa	7
Almotriptan	8
Alpha-tocopherol	8
Alprazolam	9
Alteplase	9
Amantadine	10
Amifampridine	11
Amitriptyline	12
Ammonium Tetrathiomolybdate	12
Amphetamine	13
Apixaban	14
Apomorphine	15
Aripiprazole	16
Aspirin	17
Ataluren	18
Atogepant	18
Atomoxetine	19
Atorvastatin	20
Azathioprine	20

B

Baclofen	22
Benztropine	23
Betahistine	23
Bethanechol	24
Biotin	24
Botulinum Toxin	25
Brivaracetam	26
Bromocriptine	26
Bupropion	27

C

Cabergoline	29
Candesartan Cilexetil	30
Cannabinoids	30
Capsaicin	31
Carbamazepine	31
Casimersen	32
Cenobamate	33
Chlordiazepoxide	33
Chlorpromazine	34
Cilostazol	35
Cinnarizine	36
Citicoline	36
Cladribine	37
Clobazam	37
Clomipramine	38
Clonazepam	39
Clonidine	40
Clopidogrel	41
Clozapine	41
Coenzyme Q10	42
Conivaptan	43
Cyclophosphamide	43
Cyclosporine	44

D

Dabigatran	45
Dalfampridine	46
Dantrolene	46
Darifenacin	47
Deflazacort	48
Delandistrogene Moxeparvovec	48
Desipramine	49
Dexamethasone	50
Diazepam	51
Dihydroergotamine	52
Dimenhydrinate	52
Dimethyl Fumarate	53
Dipyridamole	54
Donepezil	54
Dosulepin	55
Doxepin	55
Droxidopa (L-threo-3,4,-dihydroxyphenylserine)	56
Duloxetine	57

E

Eculizumab	58
Edaravone	59
Efgartigimod Alfa	59
Eletriptan	60
Entacapone	60
Eptinezumab	61
Erenumab	61
Escitalopram	62
Eslicarbazepine Acetate	63
Eteplirsen	63
Ethosuximide	64
Etizolam	64
Ezogabine	65

F

Felbamate	67
Fesoterodine	68
Fingolimod	68
Fludrocortisone	68
Flumazenil	69
Flunarizine	69
Fluoxetine	70
Flupirtine	71
Folic Acid	71
Fondaparinux	72
Fosphenytoin	73
Fremanezumab	74
Frovatriptan	74

G

Gabapentin (Including Gabapentin Enacarbil)	75
Galantamine	76
Galcanezumab	76
Ganciclovir	77
Gepants	78
Glatiramer Acetate	79
Givinostat	80
Golodirsen	80
Guanfacine	81

H

Haloperidol	82
Hematin	83

Hydralazine	83
Hypertonic Saline	84

I

Idebenone	85
Imipramine	85
Indomethacin	86
Inebilizumab	87
Interferon Alpha	88
Interferon Beta	88
Intravenous Immunoglobulin	89
Isoprinosine	90
Istradefylline	90

K

Ketamine	92
Ketorolac	93

L

Labetalol	94
Lacosamide	95
Lamotrigine	96
Lasmiditan	97
Lemborexant	97
Levetiracetam	98
Levodopa	99
Lidocaine	100
Low-molecular-weight Heparin	101

M

Magnesium Sulfate	102
Mannitol	103
Meclizine	104
Melatonin	104
Memantine	105
Methotrexate	106
Methylphenidate	106
Methylprednisolone	107
Mexiletine	108
Midazolam	109
Midodrine	110
Milnacipran	110

Mirabegron	111
Mirtazapine	112
Mitoxantrone	112
Modafinil	113
Morphine	113
Mycophenolate Mofetil	114

N

Naloxone	116
Naltrexone	117
Naproxen	118
Natalizumab	119
Neostigmine	121
Nicergoline	121
Nimodipine	122
Nortriptyline	123
Nusinersen	123

O

Olanzapine	125
Onasemnogene Abeparvovec	126
Ondansetron	126
Opicapone	127
Oxcarbazepine	128
Oxybutynin	129

P

Paroxetine	131
Penicillamine	132
Perampanel	133
Phenobarbital	135
Phenytoin	136
Pimavanserin	137
Piracetam	138
Pitolisant	139
Prednisolone	140
Pregabalin	140
Primidone	142
Prochlorperazine	143
Procyclidine	144
Promethazine	145
Propofol	146

Propranolol	147
Pyridoxine	147

Q

Quetiapine	149
Quinidine	150

R

Ramelteon	152
Rasagiline	153
Ravulizumab	154
Reserpine	155
Retigabine	157
Riboflavin	158
Riluzole	159
Risdiplam	159
Risperidone	161
Rituximab	162
Rivaroxaban	163
Rivastigmine	165
Ropinirole	166
Rozanolixizumab	167
Rufinamide	168

S

S1P Receptor Modulators	170
Safinamide	173
Satralizumab	174
Selegiline	174
Sertraline	175
Sodium Oxybate	176
Solifenacin	177
Sovateltide	177
Stiripentol	178
Suvorexant	178

T

Tacrolimus	180
Tafamidis	181
Tapentadol	182
Temazepam	182
Temozolomide	183
Tenecteplase	183

Teriflunomide	184
Tetrabenazine	185
Thalidomide	186
Thiamine	187
Thiocolchicoside	187
Thiopentone	188
Tiagabine	188
Ticagrelor	189
Tizanidine	190
Tocilizumab	191
Tofersen	191
Tolperisone	192
Tolterodine	192
Tolvaptan	193
Topiramate	194
Tramadol	195
Trientine	196
Trihexyphenidyl	196
Triptans	197
Trospium	198

U

Ublituximab	201
Unfractionated Heparin	202

V

Valacyclovir	204
Valbenazine	205
Valproic Acid	205
Venlafaxine	207
Verapamil	208
Vigabatrin	208

Z

Z-Drugs (Zolpidem, Zaleplon, and Zopiclone)	210
Zilucoplan	212
Zinc Acetate	212
Zonisamide	213

SECTION 2: Disease-based Catalogue of Drugs

Autoimmune Encephalitis	217
Central and Peripheral Demyelinating Disorders	217
Dementia	219

Epilepsy	219
Headache and Other Craniofacial Pain	220
Nerve and Muscle Diseases	222
Neurometabolic Disorders	223
Neuromuscular Junction Disorder	224
Neuropathic Pain	225
Parkinson's Disease	225
Sleep Disorders	226
Stroke	226
Symptomatic Treatment	227

SECTION 1

Drugs Used in Neurology

Introduction

This section arranges drugs and biologicals in an alphabetical order with a brief description of the indications, contraindications, dosage, relevant pharmacokinetics, pharmacodynamics information, drug interaction where relevant, and use in special situations and populations.

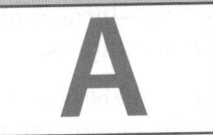

Section Outline

- Acenocoumarol
- Acetazolamide
- Acyclovir
- Aducanumab
- Albuterol
- Alemtuzumab
- Alglucosidase alfa
- Almotriptan
- Alpha-tocopherol
- Alprazolam
- Alteplase
- Amantadine
- Amifampridine
- Amitriptyline
- Ammonium tetrathiomolybdate
- Amphetamine
- Apixaban
- Apomorphine
- Aripiprazole
- Aspirin
- Ataluren
- Atogepant
- Atomoxetine
- Atorvastatin
- Azathioprine

ACENOCOUMAROL

Introduction: Coumarin derivative and vitamin K antagonist.

Pharmacodynamics: Interfere with hepatic synthesis of vitamin K-dependent clotting factors II, VII, IX, and X as well as protein C and S; depletes vitamin K reserves, which in turn reduce synthesis of active clotting factors, by competitively inhibiting subunit 1 of the multiunit K epoxide reductase complex 1 (VKOR1).

Pharmacokinetics: It has oral bioavailability of 60%. Half-life (t½) is 8–11 hours and peak plasma concentration is reached in 1–3 hours. Duration of action is 48 hours. Metabolism is by hepatic P450 enzymes CYP2C9, CYP2C19, and CYP1A2. Elimination is by 60% renal and 20% fecal route.

Use: Cerebral venous thrombosis and some cases of cardioembolic stroke.

Dose: Available in 0.5, 1, 2, 3, and 4 mg strengths. If international normalized ratio (INR) is <1.3 start at 1 mg/day. Repeat INR after 1 week. If INR is 1.4–2 add 0.5 mg/day and repeat INR after 1 week. If INR is 2.1–3 continue with current dose.

Adverse effects: Bleeding—intracranial, gastrointestinal (GI), intraocular, and hemarthrosis.

Use in special population: Elderly patients are more prone to bleeding so should be closely monitored. In pregnant women with mechanical heart valve, it is category D drug and for all other it is category X drug. Breastfeeding women may take acenocoumarol as it poses very little risk to infant. Dose reduction is needed in renal impairment and no reduction in hepatic impairment.

ACETAZOLAMIDE

Introduction: Carbonic anhydrase inhibitor.

Pharmacodynamics: Inhibits enzyme carbonic anhydrase enzyme in proximal tubules (both membrane bound and cytoplasmic forms) resulting in near complete elimination of sodium bicarbonate reabsorption. Paresthesia and somnolence may suggest its action on central nervous system (CNS). Its efficacy in epilepsy can be attributed to production of metabolic acidosis.

Pharmacokinetics: It has 100% oral bioavailability and undergoes renal excretion unchanged. t½ is 6–9 hours.

Uses: High altitude sickness, periodic paralysis, idiopathic intracranial hypertension, and catamenial seizures.

Dose: Start at 500 mg/day in two divided doses and increase up to 2 g/day. Higher doses up to 3–4 g/day tried but most of them do not tolerate the adverse effects.

Adverse effects: Somnolence, paresthesia, metabolic acidosis, bone marrow depression, allergic reactions (as they belong to sulfonamides group), and metallic taste.

Use in special population: It belongs to pregnancy category C and risk benefit consideration is advised during lactation. It is contraindicated in chronic obstructive pulmonary disease (COPD), hepatic encephalopathy, those who are taking high dose salicylates, and renal calculus (due to precipitation of calcium phosphate salts in alkaline urine). Avoid in severe renal impairment and liver cirrhosis.

ACYCLOVIR

Introduction: Acyclic guanine nucleoside analog.

Pharmacodynamics: Its action is dependent on viral thymidine kinase in herpes virus. Phosphorylation of acyclovir occurs by viral thymidine kinase. Acyclovir triphosphate is incorporated in viral deoxyribonucleic acid (DNA) and causes suicidal inhibition of viral DNA polymerase.

Pharmacokinetics: t½ is 2.5 hours and has 10–30% oral bioavailability. Renal excretion and tubular secretion are the major routes of elimination.

Uses: Highly active against herpes virus type 1. Decreasing efficacy for herpes simplex virus 2 (HSV2), varicella-zoster virus (VZV), and Epstein–Barr virus (EBV). It is least active against cytomegalovirus (CMV). EBV-related oral hairy leukoplakia may improve with acyclovir. Oral acyclovir with systemic corticosteroids appears beneficial in treating Bell's palsy in some studies; varicella zoster and herpes zoster.

Dose: Intravenous (IV) dose is 10–15 mg/kg every 8 hours for 14–21 days. Oral dose is 800 mg five times a day for 10–14 days.

Adverse effects: Nausea, vomiting, and infusion site reactions. Major adverse effects include possible precipitation of acyclovir in renal tubules and subsequent acute renal failure, encephalopathy, and thrombocytopenic purpura (TTP) rarely.

Use in special population: Dose reduction is needed in renal failure. It belongs to pregnancy category B and caution warranted while breastfeeding. Safety for oral formulation is not established in children <2 years.

ADUCANUMAB

Introduction: It is a monoclonal antibody targeting amyloid plaque aggregation. One of the controversial approval by the Food and Drug Administration (FDA) as the efficacy was not well-established. Under accelerated approval program drug was allowed in July 2021. But the manufacture had announced to withdraw the drug by January 2024 citing a "reprioritization" of the company's priorities in the Alzheimer's disease. Existing patients may receive till November 2024.

Pharmacodynamics: Human immunoglobulin G1 (IgG1) monoclonal antibody that targets aggregated forms of amyloid beta. Reduced plaque burden in a dose and time-dependent manner.

Pharmacokinetics: Half-life is 24.8 days. Maximum clinical benefits by 5 months of usage.

Uses: Alzheimer's disease at the mild cognitive impairment or mild dementia stage. Baseline MRI required prior to starting the drug. MRI should be done at 5th, 7th, 9th, and 12th infusions to detect amyloid-related imaging abnormalities (ARIAs).

Dose: Monthly infusions; available as IV formulation.

Initiation:
- Infusion 1 (at week 0) and infusion 2 (at week 4): 1 mg/kg
- Infusion 3 (at week 8) and infusion 4 (at week 12): 3 mg/kg
- Infusion 5 (at week 16) and infusion 6 (at week 20): 6 mg/kg
- Maintenance-infusion 7: 10 mg/kg every 4 weeks
- Dilution with normal saline 0.9% and given over an hour

Adverse effects: Most common adverse reactions (≥10%) include ARIAs—edema, headache, ARIA-H microhemorrhage, ARIA-H superficial siderosis, and fall. ARIAs are often asymptomatic and generally reversible with discontinuation of treatment but can cause headache, dizziness, and nausea.

Use in special population: No data is available in renal, hepatic impairment, pregnancy, or lactation.

ALBUTEROL

Introduction: It is a selective beta-2 adrenergic agonist which is approved for use in asthma and COPD.

Pharmacodynamics: Albuterol acts on beta-2 adrenergic receptors, inducing relaxation of bronchial smooth muscle and also inhibits immediate hypersensitivity mediator release, particularly from mast cells. Although albuterol also affects beta-1 adrenergic receptors, the impact is minimal, exerting little effect on the heart rate.

Pharmacokinetics: When inhaled only trace amounts of albuterol is found in bloodstream after 2–3 hours. It undergoes hepatic metabolism and renal excretion.

Uses: Primary use in neurology is in few forms of congenital myasthenic syndromes such as COLQ tail mutations, DOK7 mutation, and in agrin mutation.

Dose: The effective dose was found to be between 4 and 12 mg/day.

Adverse effects: Tremors, hypertension, cramps, and jitteriness.

Special populations: No specific recommendations in renal and liver failure. Lack of well-controlled studies for use of albuterol in pregnancy. May be used in breastfeeding.

ALEMTUZUMAB

Introduction: It is a humanized anti-CD52 monoclonal antibody.

Pharmacodynamics: It binds to CD52 protein that is found in most of the B cells, T cells, natural killer cells, and macrophages. It then induces antibody-dependent lysis of cells it has binded and produces leukopenia which can last for more than a year.

Pharmacokinetics: Initial average t½ of 1 hour, but after multiple doses, The t½ extends to 12 days and steady-state plasma concentration reaches at approximately week 6 of treatment. It is metabolized probably by proteolytic degradation.

Uses: FDA approved for relapse remitting multiple sclerosis (those who failed two other disease modifying agents).

Dose: 12 mg IV over 4 hours daily IV infusion for 5 consecutive days, then again 12 months later for 3 consecutive days. Premedication with paracetamol and chlorpheniramine advised prior to infusion.

Adverse effects: Acute infusion reactions, (myelosuppression) neutropenia, thrombocytopenia, and anemia. Patents are at risk for autoimmune hemolytic anemia, autoimmune thyroiditis, and other autoimmune diseases (probably due to immune reconstitution after a profound leukopenia). Risk of immunosuppression leads to various opportunistic infections. Particularly CMV infection is to be monitored. *Pneumocystis carinii* and herpes virus prophylaxis should be given for at least 2 months following treatment. CD4 count may be below 200 cells/μL for at least a year.

Use in special population: It is contraindicated in pregnancy. Live vaccines are not to be given to patients on treatment with alemtuzumab. Combining this drug with anticancer drugs may increase immunosuppression. No adequate data regarding its usage in renal and hepatic impairment, lactation, and pediatric safety.

ALGLUCOSIDASE ALFA

Introduction: Biosynthetic (recombinant DNA origin) form of human acid α-glucosidase (GAA).

Pharmacodynamics: It is an enzyme that catalyzes the hydrolysis of α-1,4- and α-1,6-glycosidic linkages of lysosomal glycogen. It provides an exogenous source of GAA in Pompe's disease.

Pharmacokinetics: t½ is 2–3 hours. Those who develop antibody titers of ≥12,800 at week 12 of treatment have increased clearance by about 50%.

Uses: Management of infantile-onset Pompe's disease. It is designated as orphan drug by the FDA for this condition.

Dose: Infants and children 1 month to 3.5 years of age—20 mg/kg by IV infusion once every 2 weeks. Do not exceed infusion rate > 7 mg/kg/hour.

Adverse effects: Fever, pharyngitis, respiratory distress, pneumonia, tachypnea, bronchiolitis, rash, urticaria, and other hypersensitivity reactions.

Use in special population: No recommendations at this time for special population.

ALMOTRIPTAN

Discussed under triptans.

ALPHA-TOCOPHEROL

Introduction: It also known as vitamin E, a fat-soluble vitamin. It is not produced in our body. Vitamin E is formed from photosynthetic processes of plants. It is found abundantly in avocados, wheat, green leafy vegetables, nuts, soybeans, olive oils, and sunflower oil. Alpha form of tocopherol is usually found in abundance.

Pharmacodynamics: It is a free radical scavenger and also inhibits the aggregation of platelets and monocyte adhesion.

Pharmacokinetics: It undergoes hepatic metabolism and excreted in bile and feces. It is stored in fat cells.

Uses: Ataxia with vitamin E deficiency.

Dose: Vitamin E dose ranges from 800 to 1,500 mg (or 40 mg/kg body weight in children).

Adverse effects: Nausea, headache, blurred vision, and GI upset.

Use in special population: It can be used in pregnancy and lactation. It is safe in pediatric population, renal, and hepatic failure patients.

ALPRAZOLAM

Introduction: Benzodiazepine and anxiolytic.

Pharmacodynamics: It binds to GABA-A receptor and increases the frequency of opening of chloride channels resulting in hyperpolarization and neuronal inhibition.

Pharmacokinetics: It undergoes CYP metabolism in liver. CYP3A4 inhibitors like itraconazole increase the toxicity of the drug. CYP3A4 inducer like carbamazepine decreases the levels of alprazolam. Oral bioavailability is 90%. Peak plasma concentration in 1–2 hours. Metabolites are excreted in urine. t½ is 11–12 hours. Asians have 25% greater t½ compared to Caucasians.

Uses: Anxiety and panic disorders.

Dose: 0.25–0.5 mg three times a day. Maximum is 4 mg/day for anxiety. For panic disorders 5–6 mg average dose is required and maximum dose of 10 mg may be required. Conventional and extended release are available.

Adverse effects: Withdrawal effects, drowsiness, depression, headache, constipation, diarrhea, incoordination, and fatigue.

Use in special population: In hepatic impairment and in geriatric population, use smallest effective dose. Concomitant use with opioid not recommended. It is contraindicated in pregnancy. Discontinue nursing or the drug regarding lactation.

ALTEPLASE

Introduction: Biosynthetic (recombinant DNA origin) form of human tissue-type plasminogen activator (t-PA) which is a thrombolytic agent.

Pharmacodynamics: It catalyzes the conversion of plasminogen to the proteolytic enzyme plasmin, which lyses fibrin as well as fibrinogen.

Pharmacokinetics: It is metabolized in liver and excreted in urine. It has an initial t½ of fewer than 5 minutes and a terminal t½ of 72 minutes.

Uses: Reperfusion therapy in acute ischemic stroke within a window period of 4.5 hours (after excluding bleed in the brain).

Dose: 0.9 mg/kg. 10% given as IV bolus. Rest is given as infusion over an hour. Dilute with 0.9% sodium chloride solution. Maximum dose is 90 mg.

Adverse effects: Hemorrhage (sometimes serious bleeds like intracranial hemorrhage). Increased risk of bleeding when used along with antiplatelets and anticoagulants.

Use in special population: Some of the absolute contraindications include patients with intracranial hemorrhage, neoplasm, suspected aortic dissection, active bleeding diathesis, prothrombin time (PT) INR > 1.7, uncontrolled blood pressure (BP), serious head injury, or stroke within 3 months. Safety and efficacy not established in pediatrics. Category C in pregnancy. Can be used if benefits outweigh the risk. Lactation data not available. Elimination t½ prolonged in liver failure patients hence caution warranted.

AMANTADINE

Introduction: This drug has antiparkinsonian action in addition to its use as an antiviral agent against influenza.

Pharmacodynamics: It blocks N-methyl-D-aspartate (NMDA) receptors, increases dopamine signal in striatum, and has got anticholinergic activity too.

Pharmacokinetics: It is well absorbed in gastrointestinal tract. Its half-life is 9–37 hours. There is no appreciable metabolism. The drug is eliminated by kidneys unchanged.

Uses: Can be started as an initial therapy in mild Parkinson's disease. Also used as an adjunct therapy in levodopa dose-related motor fluctuations and dyskinesia.
- *Huntington chorea*: 100 mg orally three to four times daily.
- *Multiple sclerosis-related fatigues*: 100 mg orally twice daily, increasing to 200 mg twice daily as needed.
- *Restless leg syndrome*: 100 mg orally daily, increasing to 300 mg/day as needed.
- *Traumatic brain injury*: 100 mg orally twice daily, increasing to 200 mg twice daily as needed.

Dose: 100 mg twice per day and od formulations.
- For the treatment of Parkinson disease, amantadine is also given orally at 100 mg twice daily and increased to 200 mg twice daily as needed. Dosing should begin at 100 mg once daily for patients taking other parkinsonian drugs.
- It is important not to discontinue amantadine abruptly as it can cause neuroleptic malignant syndrome (NMS)-like symptoms.

Adverse effects: Dizziness, nausea, and vomiting (mild and reversible), orthostatic hypotension, syncope, peripheral edema, dizziness, delusions, hallucinations, falls, xerostomia, and constipation. Livedo reticularis is a less common side effect. This side effect is reversible with the withdrawal of medication. Serious adverse effects include NMS, psychosis, suicidal ideation, and CNS depression.

Use in special population: It belongs to the FDA pregnancy category C. Discontinue nursing or drug during lactation. When administering amantadine, monitor BP, renal function, and mental statuses, such as depression/suicidality, and psychosis. Those with seizure disorders have to be monitored for seizure activity. Patients with heart failure require vigilance for increased water retention and lower leg edema. The clearance of amantadine greatly diminishes in elderly patients and patients with renal impairment. Therefore, dose modification merits consideration in such cases.

AMIFAMPRIDINE

Introduction: Voltage-gated potassium channel blocker. Orphan drug for Lambert–Eaton myasthenic syndrome (LEMS).

Pharmacodynamics: Blocks voltage-gated potassium channel and prevents efflux of K^+ thereby prolonging depolarization. This leads to prolonged calcium entry and enhanced acetylcholine release which improves the neuromuscular function.

Pharmacokinetics: Liver metabolism by N-acetyltransferase 2 (NAT2). Amifampridine and its inactive metabolite eliminated in urine. Orally well absorbed and peak concentration reaches in 20 minutes to 1 hour.

Uses: LEMS in children ≥ 6 years of age and in adults. To improve muscle strength (symptomatic treatment).

Dose: Begin with 15–30 mg daily in three to five divided doses. Increase 5 mg every 4 days till desired clinical response not to exceed 100 mg/day. Half the above dosing recommended in patients weighing < 45 kg.

Adverse effects: Nausea, vomiting, headache and diarrhea, paresthesia, and respiratory tract infection.

Use in special population: 5 mg in three to five divided doses in patients weighing <45 kg with hepatic impairment or creatinine clearance of 15–90 mL/min. 15 mg in three to five divided doses in patients weighing >45 kg with hepatic impairment or creatinine clearance of 15–90 mL/min. Start low dose in geriatric population. It is contraindicated in patients with history of seizures. No adequate data is available in pregnancy and lactation.

AMITRIPTYLINE

Introduction: Tricyclic antidepressant.

Pharmacodynamics: It enhances norepinephrine and serotonin neurotransmission by inhibiting their reuptake into presynaptic terminal. It also blocks histamine receptor H1, alpha-1 adrenergic, and muscarinic receptor too.

Pharmacokinetics: It undergoes liver metabolism by CYP2D6, CYP1A2, and CYP2C. Active metabolite is nortriptyline. Urine excretion of metabolites is around 25–50%. t½ is 10–50 hours. Bioavailability is 40–60%. Antidepressant effect takes 4 weeks.

Uses: Anxiety, depression, attention deficit hyperactivity disorder (ADHD), migraine, eating disorder, postherpetic neuralgia, and insomnia.

Dose: Single dose at bed time or three times a day. For >12 years 10 mg three times a day with 20 mg at bedtime for depression. In adults with depression 75 mg/day in divided doses. Maximum is 150 mg. In some patients 25–40 mg/day may be sufficient.

Adverse effects: Anticholinergic side effects include dry mouth, constipation, tachycardia, sedation, weight gain, and orthostatic hypotension, prolonged QT interval, increased suicidal tendency, and sexual dysfunction.

Use in special population: It belongs to pregnancy category C and in lactation not recommended. In children <12 years safety is not established. Avoid in geriatric age >65 years. No specific guidance in renal and liver failure. It is contraindicated in patients who had monoamine oxidase inhibitor (MAOI) in last 14 days and recovering phase of myocardial infarction. Gradually taper to avoid withdrawal effects.

AMMONIUM TETRATHIOMOLYBDATE

Introduction: Small molecule anti-copper agent to lower serum copper and not the FDA approved.

Pharmacodynamics: It reduces serum copper and improves neurological outcome in Wilson disease. It could also inhibit fibrotic process in lung. It forms a complex with copper and albumin.

Pharmacokinetics: The complex metabolized in liver.

Uses: Wilson disease.

Dose: Not available.

Adverse effects: Leukopenia.

Use in special population: Details not available.

AMPHETAMINE

Introduction: It is a racemic β-phenylisopropylamine that has CNS stimulant potential in addition to its peripheral adrenergic actions. D isomer is three to four times more potent than L isomer.

Pharmacodynamics: It stimulates the medullary respiratory center and decreases the central depression. It improves the performance of simple mental tasks, reduces fatigue, increases alertness, and ability to concentrate. It enhances analgesic effect of opioids, reduces appetite, and can postpone sleep.

The neuronal dopamine transporter (DAT) and the vesicular monoamine transporter (VMAT2) appear to be major targets of amphetamine's action and enhance release of biogenic amines from their storage terminals.

Pharmacokinetics: It is well absorbed from GI tract and therapeutic effect last 4–24 hours. It reaches maximum plasma concentration in 3 hours. Therapeutic level is 5–10 µg/dL. t½ for d-amphetamine is 9–11 hours and for l-amphetamine it is 11–13 hours. t½ increases with body weight.

Uses: Narcolepsy and ADHD.

Dose: In children aged 3–5 years, initially 2.5 mg/day. Increase by 2.5 mg weekly till adequate clinical response is attained.

In children aged ≥ 6 years initially, 5 mg once or twice daily; the daily dosage is increased in 5 mg increments at weekly intervals until the optimum response is attained. Total daily maximum dose should not exceed 40 mg. Extended release capsule preparation is also available.

Adverse effects: Irritability, weakness, nausea, vomiting, cramps, insomnia, fever, restlessness, dizziness, tremor, hyperactive reflexes, confusion, aggressiveness, changes in libido, anxiety, delirium, paranoid hallucinations, panic states, and suicidal or homicidal tendencies occur, especially in mentally ill patients. Fatigue and depression, arrhythmia, angina, hypotension, and hypertension are other adverse effects. A psychotic reaction with vivid hallucinations and paranoid delusions, often mistaken for schizophrenia, is the most common serious effect of chronic overdosage.

Use in special population: No specific dosage recommendation is available in hepatic and renal impairment. It belongs to pregnancy category C. Discontinue nursing or drug with respect to lactation. It is not recommended in children below 3 years, in patients with anorexia, insomnia, asthenia, psychopathic personality, history of drug abuse or a history of homicidal or suicidal tendencies. The abuse of amphetamine as a means of overcoming sleepiness and of increasing energy and alertness should be discouraged.

APIXABAN

Introduction: Direct factor Xa inhibitor.

Pharmacodynamics: It inhibits free and clot-associated factor Xa, which leads to reduced thrombin generation. Lack of thrombin results in poor platelet aggregation and fibrin formation is suppressed.

Pharmacokinetics: t½ is 12 hours. Bioavailability is 50% and peak concentration reaches in 1–3 hours. It is metabolized by CYP3A4 system and excreted in bile, urine, and intestine. About 27% of the drug is excreted unchanged. CYP inducers may reduce the drug levels whereas inhibitors increase drug levels.

Uses: Stroke prevention in patients with atrial fibrillation, postoperative thromboprophylaxis in patients undergoing hip or knee arthroplasty, deep venous thrombosis, and pulmonary embolism.

Dose: 5 mg twice daily is the routine dose. Dose is reduced to 2.5 mg twice daily if two out of three following criteria are present:
1. Age > 80 years
2. Body weight ≤ 60 kg
3. Serum creatinine ≥ 1.5 mg/dL

Dose can be reduced to 2.5 mg twice daily for those requiring apixaban for >6 months.

No need for coagulation parameter monitoring.

Adverse effects: Major side effect is bleeding. Intracranial bleed rates are lower than warfarin. Recombinant coagulation factor Xa called andexanet alfa is FDA approved for reversal of patients treated with apixaban who have serious bleeding.

Use in special population: It is contraindicated in atrial fibrillation patients with mechanical valves and antiphospholipid antibody syndrome. No adequate data on its use in pregnancy and lactation. No dose reduction is needed in mild hepatic impairment. Avoided in severe hepatic failure. Renal dosing as mentioned earlier.

APOMORPHINE

Introduction: This drug is a dopamine agonist and has high affinity for D4 receptors.

Pharmacodynamics: It activates dopamine receptors in nigrostriatal pathway thereby improving locomotor function.

Pharmacokinetics: Bioavailability is 100% following subcutaneous administration. Peak plasma concentrations is achieved in 10–60 minutes. Onset of action starts in 10 minutes. Therapeutic effect lasts 1 hour. Possible metabolic pathways include sulfation, N-demethylation, glucuronidation, and oxidation. t½ is 40 minutes.

Uses: FDA approved acute intermittent treatment of off period (as a rescue therapy) in Parkinson's disease.

Dose:
- Subcutaneous—2 mg initially, maximum 6 mg three or more injection per day
- Sublingual—10 mg initially, 5 mg increment, maximum 30 mg per dose up to five doses per day

Apomorphine is highly emetogenic and requires pre- and post-treatment antiemetic therapy. Oral *trimethobenzamide*, at a dose of 300 mg, three times daily, should be started 3 days prior to the initial dose of *apomorphine* and continued at least during the first 2 months of therapy.

Concomitant use of *apomorphine* with antiemetic drugs of the 5HT3 antagonist class is contraindicated as profound hypotension and loss of consciousness have occurred.

Adverse effects: Hallucination, confusion and fatigue, somnolence, sleep attacks, nausea, and orthostatic hypotension. Serious side effects of apomorphine include QT prolongation, injection site reactions, and the development of a pattern of abuse characterized by increasingly frequent dosing leading to hallucinations, dyskinesia, and abnormal behavior. The sublingual formulation can cause oral sores.

Use in special population: No dose adjustment is needed in hepatic impairment. In renal failure, start at lower dose (1 mg).

ARIPIPRAZOLE

Introduction: Quinolinone antipsychotic; fewer adverse effects than older antipsychotics.

Pharmacodynamics: It is a partial agonist at D2 receptors. Higher affinity for D2 than 5HT2A receptors. Competes with dopamine in striatum and reduces hyperdopaminergic activity. It also has agonist activity in prefrontal cortex enhancing dopaminergic transmission. This dual action is helpful in treating both positive and negative symptoms of schizophrenia.

Pharmacokinetics: It reaches maximum concentration in 3-5 hours. It undergoes CYP2D6 and 3A4 metabolism to produce active metabolite and dehydroaripiprazole. t½ for aripiprazole is 75 hours and for dehydroaripiprazole it is 94 hours.

Uses: Only antipsychotic FDA approved for the treatment of Tourette disorder; irritability associated with autism in child and adolescent patients (ages 5-16 years); symptomatic management of psychosis in patients with schizophrenia and monotherapy or adjunctive therapy for acute manic episodes associated with bipolar disorder.

Dose:
- Tourette dose—start at doses of 2 mg/day and increase (if needed) to a maximum of 10 mg/day for those weighing <50 kg or to 20 mg/day if weighing 50 kg or more.
- Autism—start at 2 mg/day, 5-10 mg is the usual maintenance dose, maximum to a dose of 15 mg.
- Double the dose in 1-2 weeks if strong CYP3A4 inducers are used along. Reduce the usual dose to half if used along with strong CYP2D6 inhibitors.

Adverse effects: Nausea, vomiting, akathisia, and compulsive behaviors. Less risk of metabolic problems such as syndrome of inappropriate antidiuretic hormone secretion (SIADH), hyperglycemia, weight gain, hyperprolactinemia, and extrapyramidal side effects compared to older antipsychotics. Serious side effects include NMS.

Use in special population: It belongs to pregnancy category C. Discontinue nursing or drug regarding lactation. No dose adjustment is required in severe hepatic or even severe renal failure.

ASPIRIN

Introduction: Nonsteroidal anti-inflammatory drug (NSAID), antiplatelet agent, and salicylic acid.

Pharmacodynamics: In platelets cyclooxygenase (COX-1) catalyzes the formation of thromboxane A2 which is a platelet aggregator and vasoconstrictor. Aspirin inhibits COX-1 by acetylating serine residue near the active site thereby preventing formation of thromboxane A2. The effect of aspirin is permanent on platelets and lasts till the lifetime of platelets (7–10 days). Cumulative effect on platelet inhibition happens with repeated dosing.

Pharmacokinetics: It is metabolized to salicylic acid. It is orally well absorbed and reaches peak concentration in 1–2 hours. Unhydrolyzed aspirin subsequently undergoes hydrolysis by esterases mainly in the liver. Salicylic acid is metabolized by liver microsomal system and predominantly eliminated by renal excretion. t½ is 3 hours at 300 mg of aspirin.

Uses: Secondary prevention of ischemic stroke, ischemic heart disease, and peripheral arterial disease.

Dose: 75 mg/day is effective for antiplatelet action. Dose ranges from 50 to 325 mg. Higher doses increase the risk of toxicity. In children 3–5 mg/kg is given for ischemic stroke for 2 years.

Adverse effects: GI toxicity includes irritation, bleeding, tinnitus, bronchospasm, ulcer, and perforation risk of Reye syndrome if used in children with varicella and influenza infections. Increases bleeding time.

Use in special population: It is contraindicated in asthma, urticarial, and hypersensitivity to NSAIDs. Lactation is not recommended in mothers taking aspirin. Used only if there is benefit over risk. Lowest possible dose is preferred. Use in second trimester can cause fetal renal dysfunction. Use in 30 or more weeks pregnant women may cause premature closure of ductus arteriosus of the fetus. Avoid in severe hepatic or renal impairment.

ATALUREN

Introduction: Antisense oligonucleotide used in nonsense mutation Duchenne muscular dystrophy (nmDMD). European medicine agency (EMA) gave conditional approval in 2014 that the efficacy must be confirmed by 2021. The US FDA rejected this drug application in 2017 after reviewing the data. At the time of writing this book, the EMA has not renewed the drug authorization by 2024.

Pharmacodynamics: Ataluren acts at ribosomal translational machinery. It enables the read through of premature stop codon due to nonsense mutation of messenger ribonucleic acid (mRNA) and thereby promoting the production of functional dystrophin protein.

Pharmacokinetics: It is metabolized by conjugation via uridine diphosphate glucuronosyltransferase (UGT) enzymes, predominantly UGT1A9 in liver and intestine. Peak plasma concentration is achieved in 1.5 hours.

Uses: Ambulant children with nmDMD aged ≥ 5 years.

Dose: Morning and mid-day dose is 10 mg/kg whereas night dose is 20 mg/kg (total 40 mg/kg/day). Oral granules are to be taken by mouth after mixing them with liquid or semisolid food (such as yogurt).

Adverse effects: Nausea, vomiting, and diarrhea.

Use in special population: Data not available.

ATOGEPANT

Introduction: Small molecule calcitonin gene-related peptide (CGRP) receptor antagonist.

Pharmacodynamics: CGRP has a role in multiple pathophysiologic mechanisms underlying migraine attacks. CGRP is a neuropeptide released in trigeminocervical complex system that plays a major role in cerebral vessels vasodilation and pain modulation. It binds to CGRP receptors with high affinity, blocking the binding of CGRP to the receptor, and preventing subsequent receptor activation.

Pharmacokinetics: It takes 1–2 hours to reach maximum plasma concentration. t½ is 11 hours. It is metabolized in liver by CYP3A4 system and majority of drug excreted in feces. Strong CYP3A4 inhibitors increase levels of atogepant.

Use: For episodic and chronic migraine prevention.

Dose: Usual dose is 60 mg oral daily; for patients prone for constipation use 30 mg. Use 10 mg daily if CYP3A4 strong inhibitors are used for episodic prevention. For chronic prevention do not use CYP3A4 strong inhibitors along with atogepant.

Adverse effects: Fatigue, somnolence, nausea, and constipation.

Use in special population: Dosage adjustment is not needed in mild to moderate renal failure. In severe renal failure, use 10 mg daily. In mild to moderate liver disease, no dose adjustment is needed. Avoid in severe liver disease. Data on pregnancy, lactation, and pediatric safety is inadequate.

ATOMOXETINE

Introduction: Serotonin-norepinephrine reuptake inhibitors (SNRIs).

Pharmacodynamics: SNRI that inhibits the reuptake of both norepinephrine and serotonin.

Pharmacokinetics: It is metabolized in liver by CYP2D6 to an equipotent metabolite (4-hydroxyatomoxetine). It is orally well absorbed. Poor metabolizers have 94% bioavailability and t½ of 22 hours. CYP2C19 substrate metabolizers have 63% oral bioavailability and t½ of 5 hours. Peak concentration is reached in 1–2 hours.

Uses: Treatment of ADHD in children ≥ 6 years.

Dose:
- *Children and adolescents weighing ≤70 kg*: Initially, approximately 0.5 mg/kg daily. Increase dosage after ≥3 days to target dosage of approximately 1.2 mg/kg daily (do not exceed 100 mg daily).
- *Children and adolescents weighing >70 kg*: Initially, 40 mg daily. Increase dosage after ≥3 days to target dosage of approximately 80 mg daily.

Adverse effects: Increase suicidal risk, psychotic symptoms in children, sudden death in structural heart disease, and hepatic injury. Common adverse effects are abdominal pain, decreased appetite, vomiting, somnolence, nausea, fatigue, irritability, and dizziness in children. In adults, dry mouth, nausea, insomnia, decreased appetite, constipation, fatigue, erectile dysfunction, hot flush, urinary hesitation and/or retention, and dysmenorrhea.

Use in special population: Reduce dose to 50% in moderate hepatic failure and 75% in severe liver dysfunction. 2 weeks gap is needed between MAOI and atomoxetine. It is contraindicated in angle closure glaucoma. It belongs to pregnancy category C. Caution while nursing. Safety is not established in children < 6 years.

ATORVASTATIN

Introduction: HMG-CoA reductase inhibitors.

Pharmacodynamics: Competitively and selectively inhibits HMG-CoA reductase leading to reduction in hepatic cholesterol synthesis. It also has anti-inflammatory activity and cause regression or slows progression of atherosclerosis in coronary and carotid arteries. It reduces low-density lipoprotein (LDL), very low-density lipoprotein (VLDL), total cholesterol, and increases high-density lipoprotein (HDL).

Pharmacokinetics: It is rapidly absorbed from gut but undergoes extensive first pass metabolism. Absolute bioavailability is only 14%. Therapeutic effect starts at 2 weeks and maximum at 4 weeks. It is metabolized in the liver, mainly by CYP3A4. t½ is approximately 14 hours. Drug is eliminated via feces.

Uses: Dyslipidemia, reduction of coronary and cerebro-vascular events.

Dose: 10–80 mg.

Adverse effects: Arthralgia, muscle spasms, myalgia, insomnia, diarrhea, urinary tract infection, and dyspepsia. Rhabdomyolysis with acute renal failure secondary to myoglobinuria and immune-mediated necrotizing myopathy (IMNM) are reported rarely.

Use in special population: No dose adjustment is required in renal failure. Caution warranted in hepatic impairment even though no guideline is given. It is better to avoid in pregnancy. Discontinue nursing or drug during lactation. It is contraindicated in active liver disease.

AZATHIOPRINE

Introduction: This purine antimetabolite is an imidazolyl derivative of 6-mercaptopurine (6 MP).

Pharmacodynamics: Azathioprine is converted to 6 MP nonenzymatically. 6 MP is metabolized to 6-thio-GMP and incorporated into DNA thereby preventing cell proliferation inhibiting variety of lymphocyte functions.

Pharmacokinetics: It is orally well absorbed and peak plasma concentration is expected within 1–2 hours of drug intake. It undergoes methylation and oxidation in liver and erythrocytes. t½ of azathioprine and 6 MP are 10 minutes and 1 hour, respectively. Allopurinol increases toxicity of the drug as it inhibits xanthine oxidase which also metabolizes azathioprine metabolites.

Uses: Licensed in polymyositis, dermatomyositis, and systemic lupus erythematosus. Other off label indications include myasthenia gravis, LEMS, chronic inflammatory demyelinating polyneuropathy, multifocal motor neuropathy, multiple sclerosis, neuromyelitis optica, neurosarcoidosis, cerebral vasculitis, and autoimmune encephalitis.

Dose: Initial starting dose is 0.5 mg/kg/day to 1 mg/kg/day. Over 3 weeks dose is increased to 2–2.5 mg/kg/day. Measuring thiopurine methyltransferase (TPMT) levels before starting drug is recommended. Those who have intermediate levels of TPMT activity, 1 mg/kg/day is recommended. 2 mg/kg/day is for those with high TPMT levels. It can take up to 18 months for the therapeutic effect.

Adverse effects: Bone marrow suppression and hepatotoxicity. Fortnightly leukocyte counts and liver function tests are essential when starting azathioprine. Once on a stable dose for 6 weeks, reduce the frequency to monthly for 3 months and then every 12 weeks while continuing azathioprine. Viral infections such as human immunodeficiency virus (HIV), HSV, and VZV to be ruled out before starting azathioprine.

Use in special population: Azathioprine is safe in pregnancy and breastfeeding, and probably has a low long-term malignancy risk. Drug is contraindicated in people with complete TPMT deficiency. Administer pneumococcal vaccine before starting azathioprine and the influenza vaccine annually.

B

Section Outline

- Baclofen
- Benztropine
- Betahistine
- Bethanechol
- Biotin
- Botulinum toxin
- Brivaracetam
- Bromocriptine
- Bupropion

BACLOFEN

Introduction: GABA-B receptor agonist.

Pharmacodynamics: It inhibits release of excitatory neurotransmitter at presynaptic neurons and facilitates inhibitory signals from postsynaptic neurons in brain and spinal cord thereby relieving spasticity.

Pharmacokinetics: Oral bioavailability is 70%. Peak concentration occurs in 1 hour and half-life (t½) is 3.75 hours. Majority of the drug is excreted in urine 70%.

Uses: Intrathecal delivery using catheter and pump for spasticity as it reduces the sedation side effect. Risk of central nervous system (CNS) depression is high on abrupt withdrawal. It can be used off label for alcohol use disorder to achieve abstinence or maintain abstinence. Risk of sedation is higher if combined with alcohol.

Dose: Oral dose at 5–10 mg/day initially and increase gradually up to 200 mg/day.

Adverse effects: Fatigue, weakness, drowsiness, and dizziness for oral baclofen. For intrathecal dizziness, nausea, hypotension, and headache are possible adverse effects.

Use in special population: It belongs to category C in pregnancy. Breastfeeding is not recommended when mother takes oral baclofen. For mothers receiving intrathecal baclofen nursing is advised if benefits outweigh risk. Dose is increased gradually in elderly. Dose reduction is needed in renal failure.

BENZTROPINE

Introduction: Synthetic muscarinic receptor antagonist; structural resemblance with diphenhydramine, and atropine.

Pharmacodynamics: It antagonizes acetylcholine and histamine receptors. It reduces central cholinergic activity which helps in alleviating Parkinson symptoms.

Pharmacokinetics: It undergoes hepatic metabolism and excreted in bile and urine.

Uses: The Food and Drug Administration (FDA) approved as an adjunctive therapy for various forms of parkinsonism, including idiopathic and postencephalitic parkinsonism and drug-induced dystonia.

Dose: Oral, intravenous (IV), and intramuscular (IM) formulations are available. Oral drug is started at 0.5 mg/day and increase up to 6 mg/day. 1 mg is given IV or IM for acute dystonic reaction.

Adverse effects: Dry mouth, blurred vision, constipation, hallucination, delirium, and tachycardia.

Use in special population: No adequate data is available in renal, hepatic, pregnancy, and lactation patients. Geriatric population are vulnerable to anticholinergic side effects such as delirium and confusion. Hence, lower dose preferred in geriatric patients.

BETAHISTINE

Introduction: Antivertigo agent in Ménière's disease though not approved in USA, it is widely used in UK and European countries.

Pharmacodynamics: Histamine H1 weak agonist and H3 antagonist causing vasodilation and increasing vestibulocochlear blood flow and reducing endolymphatic pressure.

Pharmacokinetics: It is metabolized primarily into the inactive metabolite 2-pyridylacetic acid and excreted in urine predominantly. Peak concentration is attained in 1 hour. t½ is 3–4 hours.

Uses: Used in Ménière's disease and any vertigo of vestibular origin.

Dose: Available in 8, 16, and 24 mg. Initial dose is 8–16 mg three times a day. Maximum dose is 24–48 mg/day.

Adverse effects: Nausea, vomiting, somnolence, and anaphylaxis.

Use in special population: It is contraindicated in asthma, urticaria, and peptic ulcer disease.

BETHANECHOL

Introduction: Synthetic choline derivative and beta-methyl analog of carbachol that has predominantly muscarinic activity on gut motility and bladder. It lacks nicotinic activity and not susceptible to hydrolysis by acetylcholinesterase.

Pharmacodynamics: It exerts its effects by directly stimulating the muscarinic receptors (M1, M2, M3, M4, and M5) of the parasympathetic nervous system.

Pharmacokinetics: It has poor oral bioavailability. Action lasts 1 hour and effect starts in 30 minutes and peaks at 60–90 minutes. Metabolism and elimination not much known.

Uses: It helps in emptying bladder in the absence of obstruction of the urinary tract. So it is used in postoperative urinary retention, diabetic autonomic neuropathy, and certain cases of chronic hypotonic, myogenic, or neurogenic bladder. It was also previously used to treat gastrointestinal motility disorders such as gastroparesis and adynamic ileus.

Dose: 10–50 mg three to four times a day, taken 1–2 hours before meals to avoid nausea.

Adverse effects: Common adverse effects include profuse sweating, diarrhea, hypotension cramps, and nausea.

Use in special population: Contraindicated in asthma, hyperthyroidism (may precipitate atrial fibrillation), epilepsy patients, urinary and gastrointestinal obstruction, heart disease with hypotension, and bradycardia. Pregnancy and lactation studies are lacking. Safety and effectiveness not established in pediatric population.

BIOTIN

Introduction: It is also called as vitamin H or B7.

Pharmacodynamics: It has a role in cell signaling and epigenetic regulation. It is a coenzyme for multiple carboxylases (pyruvate carboxylase, propionyl-CoA carboxylase, methylcrotonyl CoA carboxylase, and acetyl CoA carboxylase) in humans.

Pharmacokinetics: It is widely protein bound. Metabolized by liver and excreted in kidneys.

Uses: Biotinidase deficiency (developmental delay, ataxia, and seizures in neonates), brittle hair, patients on long-term anticonvulsants.

Egg yolk, liver, cereals, and vegetables such as spinach, mushroom, and rice are natural sources of biotin.

Dose: 5–35 µg/day. Oral tablet form comes in 10, 50, and 100 µg.

Adverse effects: Abdominal pain.

Use in special population: Patients on long-term anticonvulsants, pregnant, and lactating mothers require biotin supplementation.

BOTULINUM TOXIN

Introduction: Botulinum toxin is a peripherally acting antispasticity agent. AbobotulinumtoxinA, incobotulinumtoxinA, onabotulinumtoxinA, prabotulinumtoxinA-xvfs, and rimabotulinumtoxinB are the various nonequivalent preparations which act by blocking acetylcholine release.

Pharmacodynamics: It binds to presynaptic cholinergic nerve terminal and SNARE protein is cleaved into fragments thereby preventing vesicular release of acetylcholine. This results in skeletal muscle paralysis and also inhibition of sympathetic and parasympathetic synapses. The effect lasts for few weeks to 3 months.

Pharmacokinetics: Limited data in humans.

Uses: Conditions such as dystonias, spasticity of extremities, hemifacial spasm, blepharospasm, overactive bladder, migraine prophylaxis, anal sphincter disorders, and primary hyperhidrosis benefit from local injection of botulinum toxin. It is also used cosmetically for a wrinkle-free face.

Dose: Varies based on the preparation used. Dose is individualized and lowest starting dose is recommended. It can be repeated not <12 weeks to avoid neutralizing antibody formation.

Adverse effects: Hypersensitivity reactions, distant migration from the injection site may cause dysphagia, respiratory paralysis as in cervical dystonia. Antitoxin is available but may not reverse the weakness in already affected muscles. It stabilizes and prevents further worsening.

Use in special population: Not recommended in pregnancy as the studies are not available in humans, but caused abortions and malformations in animals.

Breastfeeding can be considered if benefits outweigh risks.

Use with caution in patients with neuromuscular disorders such as amyotrophic lateral sclerosis and myasthenia gravis.

BRIVARACETAM

Introduction: Racetam analog.

Pharmacodynamics: Mechanism by which synaptic vesicle protein 2A (SV2A) exerts antiseizure activity is less clear. May involve ligand-mediated SV2A conformational changes that convey some seizure protective effects. It binds with high selectivity to the SV2A with 15- to 30-fold higher affinity than levetiracetam.

Pharmacokinetics: Brivaracetam is more lipophilic and has greater brain-permeability than levetiracetam, due to its propyl side chain. Peak concentration is attained in 0.5–2 hours. It has good oral bioavailability and undergoes liver metabolism by CYP2C19 and CYP2C9. t½ is 9 hours.

Use: FDA approved in 2016 as an adjunctive therapy for focal-onset seizures in patients with epilepsy aged 16 years and older. From 2021 FDA approved IV, oral, and tablet form usage in children 1 month and older.

Dose: IV, oral, and tablet forms are available. The recommended initial dose for brivaracetam is 50 mg twice daily, based on patient response and tolerability may be adjusted to either 25 mg twice daily or 100 mg twice daily.

Adverse effects: Nausea, vomiting sedation, and dizziness.

Use in special population: In liver disease, half the dose reduction is needed. No dose change in renal failure. It belongs to pregnancy category C and no data is available on lactation.

BROMOCRIPTINE

Introduction: Semisynthetic ergot alkaloid that acts as a dopamine receptor agonist.

Pharmacodynamics: Acts on D2 receptor of anterior pituitary lactotropes and enhances dopamine transmission that results in reduced gene expression and reduced exocytosis of prolactin.

Pharmacokinetics: It has short t½ (2–8 hours) and undergoes extensive first pass metabolism; only 7% reaches systemic circulation.

Uses: Hyperprolactinemia (most often due to prolactinoma), type 2 diabetes for glycemic control, acromegaly, and Parkinson disease. Off-label uses include peripartum cardiomyopathy and neuroleptic malignant syndrome.

Dose: 1.25–2.5 mg/day to begin with. Then increase 2.5 mg every 2–7 days till desired response. Usual therapeutic dose is 2.5–15 mg/day (in divided doses). For Parkinson disease higher doses may be required (30–100 mg/day). For diabetes mellitus a quick release (Cycloset) preparation of dose 0.8 mg/day is used. Increment weekly by 0.8 mg till glycemic control is achieved or to a maximum of 4.8 mg is advised.

Adverse effects: Common side effects include nausea, vomiting, dizziness, hypotension, and headache. CNS side effects are psychosis, hallucinations, nightmares, and insomnia. Hence, start at a low dose at bedtime with a snack.

Use in special population: Use low dose when using concomitantly with CYP3A4 inhibitors. It is contraindicated in syncope, psychosis, and type 1 diabetes mellitus. Dose reduction needed in hepatic impairment as the liver is primary metabolizing organ for this drug. No dose reduction is needed in renal failure. It is not recommended in pregnancy and lactation (can suppress lactation).

BUPROPION

Introduction: It contains beta-phenylethylamine as chemical backbone.

Pharmacodynamics: It increases the dopaminergic and noradrenergic transmission by inhibiting reuptake by dopamine and norepinephrine transporter. It also probably enhances presynaptic transmission.

Pharmacokinetics: It undergoes hepatic metabolism by CYP2D6. Plasma concentration peaks in 5 hours after extended release preparation. It has good oral bioavailability. Metabolites are excreted in urine. t½ is 14 hours.

Uses: Major depression, seasonal depressive disorder, and smoking cessation. Off-label use in neuropathic pain, weight loss, and attention deficit hyperactivity disorder (ADHD).

Dose: Begin with 150 mg extended release once daily in morning and increase to 150 mg twice on 4th day. Available in 150, 300, and 450 mg extended release preparation. 150 mg extended release every other day in moderate to severe hepatic impairment. 150 mg extended release every 3 days in patients undergoing hemodialysis.

Adverse effects: Common side effects include dizziness, nausea, vomiting, dry mouth, hyperhidrosis, and tremor. Fewer sexual side effects compared to other antidepressants and causes weight gain. It is contraindicated in eating disorders, epilepsy (dose-dependent increase in seizures), alcohol, benzodiazepine withdrawal, and monoamine oxidase (MAO) inhibitors.

It may increase suicide risk in young adults. Mania in bipolar disorder, neuropsychiatric disturbances like hallucination, panic attacks, anxiety, irritability, and aggression was noted when used in smoking cessation purpose.

Use in special population: Safety and efficacy is not established in pediatric population. Only if benefit outweighs risk, it is advised to use in pregnancy. It is secreted in breast milk and some postmarketing surveillance reports seizures in breastfed infants though causal relationship was not established.

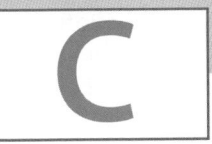

Section Outline

- Cabergoline
- Candesartan cilexetil
- Cannabinoids
- Capsaicin
- Carbamazepine
- Casimersen
- Cenobamate
- Chlordiazepoxide
- Chlorpromazine
- Cilostazol
- Cinnarizine
- Citicoline
- Cladribine
- Clobazam
- Clomipramine
- Clonazepam
- Clonidine
- Clopidogrel
- Clozapine
- Coenzyme Q10
- Conivaptan
- Cyclophosphamide
- Cyclosporine

CABERGOLINE

Introduction: Ergot derivative, more selective for D2 dopamine receptor than bromocriptine.

Pharmacodynamics: It acts on D2 receptor of anterior pituitary lactotropes and enhances dopamine transmission that results in reduced gene expression and reduced exocytosis of prolactin.

Pharmacokinetics: It has longer half-life (t½) of 65 hours and undergoes extensive first pass metabolism.

Uses: Preferred drug for hyperprolactinemia as it has good efficacy and fewer adverse effects.

Dose: Start at 0.25 mg twice per week or 0.5 mg per week. Increase to a dose of 1.5–2 mg two times a week gradually (increase once in every 4 weeks).

Adverse effects: Nausea and vomiting occur in less number of patients when compared with bromocriptine. Hypotension and dizziness can occur. Valvular heart disease are at only higher doses (>2 mg/week).

Use in special population: It is contraindicated in patients with valvular heart diseases and fibrotic disorders. Not recommended in pregnancy and lactation (interference with lactation). Dose reduction may be needed in severe hepatic impairment. No adjustment is required in renal failure. Pediatric safety and efficacy is not established.

CANDESARTAN CILEXETIL

Introduction: It is an inactive ester prodrug which is converted to active metabolite candesartan.

Pharmacodynamics: Angiotensin receptor blocker competitively inhibiting AT1 receptor activation. By preventing vasoconstriction in cerebral vessel smooth muscles it may prevent migraine attacks.

Pharmacokinetics: t½ is 9 hours. Peak plasma concentration is achieved in 3–4 hours after oral ingestion. Two-thirds of the drug is eliminated by biliary excretion and one-third by renal excretion.

Uses: Apart from its antihypertensive effect, it can be used for migraine prevention where it may be effective.

Dose: Usual dose is 8–16 mg/day in one or two divided doses. Maximum is 32 mg/day.

Adverse effects: Dizziness, pharyngitis, rhinitis, hyperkalemia, hypotension, and anaphylactic reactions.

Use in special population: Lower doses are recommended for moderate to severe hepatic and renal impairment. It belongs to pregnancy category D and must not be used in pregnancy. Data on lactation is not available.

CANNABINOIDS

Introduction: It is a phytocannabinoid derivative from the plant *Cannabis sativa* and lacks the psychoactive effect of tetrahydrocannabinol.

Pharmacodynamics: The mechanism behind antiseizure efficacy is not known. Postulated mechanisms include activation of TRPV1 (vanilloid receptor), 5HT1A receptor and inhibition of equilibrative nucleoside transporter 1 (ENT-1) to regulate adenosine tone.

Pharmacokinetics: It is highly lipophilic and binds to adipose tissue. It has a long t½ of 18–32 hours. Oral absorption is better after a fatty meal. It is metabolized by cytochrome p450 enzymes in liver and intestine. When used with antiepileptics that induce CYP (carbamazepine and phenytoin) levels of cannabinoids (CBD) decrease whereas when used with sodium valproate (CYP inhibitor) CBD levels may increase.

Uses: Seizures associated with Lennox–Gastaut syndrome, Dravet syndrome, and tuberous sclerosis complex in patients who are 1 year of age and older.

Dose: To start 2.5 mg/kg twice a day; after 1 week, may increase to maintenance dose of 5 mg/kg twice daily.

Adverse effects: Diarrhea, fatigue, vomiting, and drowsiness.

Use in special population: Liver enzymes should be monitored at 1st, 3rd, and 6th month after starting the drug. Dose reduction is needed in moderate (start at 2.5 mg/kg/day and maintain at 5 mg/kg/day) to severe hepatic failure (start at 1.25 mg/kg than maintain at 2–4 mg/kg). No dose adjustment required in renal failure.

CAPSAICIN

Introduction: Chilli pepper extract.

Pharmacodynamics: TRPV1 agonist. Acting on TRPV1 causes depolarization and signals propagate to cord and brain. It desensitizes sensory afferent nerve fibers. Repeated application depletes substance P which is a chemomediator for pain.

Pharmacokinetics: t½ is 1.64 hours.

Uses: Postherpetic neuralgia, neuropathic pain, pruritus, burning mouth pain

Dose: 0.025% topical gel in combination with diclofenac and gabantin, 8% topical patch are available formulation.

Adverse effects: Local site reaction—erythema, edema and pruritus. Sometimes nausea, vomiting, and hypertension.

Use in special population: Contraindicated in asthma.

CARBAMAZEPINE

Introduction: Iminostilbene; approved for use in epilepsy in 1974.

Pharmacodynamics: It competitively inhibits fast voltage-gated sodium channels, stabilizing the inactivated state and the sodium-dependent release of neurotransmitters. Reduces the high-frequency neuronal firing.

Pharmacokinetics: It has good oral bioavailability and metabolized in liver by CYP3A4 enzymes (vulnerable to drug interactions). Carbamazepine-10,11-epoxide is one of the significant metabolite implicated in some of the drug's side effect. Concomitant use of valproate increases toxicity due to accumulation of epoxide metabolite. It is a strong inducer of CYP. CYP inhibitors increase levels of the drug. It induces its own metabolism (autoinduction) resulting in shorter t½ and low-serum levels. Hence, lower dose is initiated first. t½ is 25–65 hours initially; 12–17 hours with multiple dosing.

Uses: IV form available from 2016. Usually oral form is used. It is not a good choice in immunoglobulin E (IgE) syndromes. It is effective against focal seizures and generalized tonic–clonic seizures but it may exacerbate absence, myoclonic, and atonic seizures. It is the FDA approved for trigeminal neuralgia, acute mania and bipolar disorder. Rebound seizures can occur on abrupt withdrawal. It also used as an off-label treatment for neuropathic pain.

Dose: Initial dose is 100 mg two times a day or 200 mg at bedtime. Increase 200 mg every 3 days to a target total daily dosage of 400–800 mg in two divided doses. Therapeutic level is 4–12 mg/L.

Adverse effects: Sedation, nausea, headache, dizziness, fatigue, ataxia, diplopia, nystagmus, tremor, hyponatremia, decreased bone weight, and rarely aplastic anemia.

Use in special population: HLA-B*1502 allele in individuals of Asian descent are vulnerable to serious idiosyncratic drug reactions such as Stevens–Johnson syndrome (SJS) and toxic epidermal necrolysis (TEN). Hence, routine testing of the allele prior to starting the drug is recommended. Monitor complete blood count (CBC) and liver function test (LFT) before therapy, at 2nd month and every 6–12 months. It causes fetal harm and belongs to the FDA pregnancy category D. Discontinue nursing or the drug during lactation period. Use in renal failure and hepatic failure is based on risk benefit ratio.

CASIMERSEN

Introduction: Antisense oligonucleotide (ASO), indicated in Duchenne muscular dystrophy (DMD) patients who have mutation that is amenable to exon 45 skipping. Increases dystrophin production.

Pharmacodynamics: This ASO binds to pre-messenger ribonucleic acid (mRNA) transcript and hides exon 45 from the RNA splicing machinery. This action results in restoring the reading frame thereby producing a functional protein.

Pharmacokinetics: Elimination t½ was 3.5 hours. It is mostly excreted unchanged in the urine.

Uses: DMD with mutation amenable to exon 45 skipping.

Dose: It is available as 2 mL vial which contains 100 mg. Standard dose is 30 mg/kg of bodyweight given once weekly IV over 35–60 minutes.

Adverse effects: Fever, headache, cough, arthralgia, and upper respiratory tract.

Use in special population: Prior renal function testing (preferably cystatin C and urine dipstick, urine protein creatinine ratio) is advised. Monitor the same every 3 months. No data in pregnancy, lactation, renal, and hepatic impairment.

CENOBAMATE

Introduction: It is a tetrazole carbamate derivative.

Pharmacodynamics: Proposed mechanism of action includes enhancement of inactivation of both fast and slow sodium channel and persistent sodium current inhibition. It is also a positive allosteric regulator of GABA-A.

Pharmacokinetics: It undergoes liver metabolism by CYP enzymes. It has a t½ of 30–76 hours and reaches peak plasma concentration in 1–4 hours. It also induces CYP hence drug-drug interaction potential is high.

Uses: Focal seizures in adults both as a monotherapy and as an add-on agent.

Dose: Initial dose is 12.5 mg/day for the first 2 weeks. Increase to 50 mg for the next 2 weeks. Then every 2 weeks increment dose of 50 mg. Maximum dose is 200–400 mg/day. Oral formulation is available and given once daily.

Adverse effects: Shortens QT interval, nausea, somnolence, diplopia, and fatigue. Drug reaction with eosinophilia and systemic symptoms (DRESS) if dose escalated rapidly.

Use in special population: Maximum dose is 200 in mild to moderate liver disease and contraindicated in severe disease. No human data in children, pregnancy, and lactation.

CHLORDIAZEPOXIDE

Introduction: It is a long-acting and self-tapering (due to active metabolites) benzodiazepine.

Pharmacodynamics: It binds to GABA-A receptor and increases the frequency of opening of chloride channels resulting in hyperpolarization and neuronal inhibition.

Pharmacokinetics: Drug is metabolized in the liver by hydroxylation and conjugation. Major active metabolites include demoxepam, desmethylchlordiazepoxide, desmethyldiazepam, and oxazepam. t½ is 5–30 hours. It is quite longer for metabolites. Inactive metabolites are excreted in urine.

Uses: Alcohol withdrawal, anxiety, and preoperative anxiolysis. It is available as fixed combination with clidinium bromide in functional gastrointestinal (GI) disorders like irritable bowel syndrome (IBS).

Dose:
- In alcohol withdrawal 50–100 mg initially, not to exceed 300 mg/day to control agitation. Taper to lowest dose after agitation is controlled.
- For mild to moderate anxiety 5–10 mg three to four times a day.
- For severe anxiety 20–25 mg three to four times a day.
- Combination with amitriptyline is also available (25 mg amitriptyline and 10 mg chlordiazepoxide).

Adverse effects: Confusion, ataxia, and drowsiness.

Use in special population: Dose reduction is needed in hepatic impairment. No dose reduction is needed in renal failure. In geriatric, use smallest effective dose. Do not use with opioids. No safety data is available below 6 years. It belongs to pregnancy category D. Discontinue nursing or drug during lactation.

CHLORPROMAZINE

Introduction: Propylamine-derivative phenothiazine and first-generation antipsychotic.

Pharmacodynamics: D2 blocker.

Pharmacokinetics: It reaches maximum plasma concentration within 1.4–2 hours. Bioavailability is based on dose used (8–14% with 25 mg, 18–34% with 100 mg). t½ is 11–15 hours (range, 8–33 hours with chronic dosing). It undergoes CYP2D6 metabolism. Strong CYP1A2 and CYP2D6 inhibitors will increase drug levels by as much as 38% and 70%, respectively.

Uses: Symptomatic management of psychotic disorders, intractable hiccup, nausea and vomiting, disruptive behavior in attention deficit hyperactivity disorder (ADHD), and acute intermittent porphyria. Initial therapeutic response in 1-4 weeks. Optimum response in 6 months.

Dose: 0.55 mg/kg every 4-6 hours as necessary for children from 6 months to 12 years. Parenteral and oral forms are available. Initiate oral in adults in dose of 25 mg TDS. Then increase by 20-50 mg twice weekly till desired response.

Adverse effects: Acute dystonia, akathisia, parkinsonism, neuroleptic malignant syndrome (NMS), rabbit syndrome, tardive dyskinesia, hyperprolactinemia, leukopenia and neutropenia, cholestatic jaundice, and anticholinergic side effects such as dry mouth, constipation and orthostatic hypotension.

Use in special population: It should not be used in children <6 months of age. It is contraindicated in comatose states and in patients who are on huge doses of central nervous system (CNS) depressants. It belongs to pregnancy category C. Discontinue nursing or drug during lactation.

CILOSTAZOL

Introduction: Quinolinone derivative that acts as platelet aggregation inhibitor.

Pharmacodynamics: Phosphodiesterase (PDE) type 3 inhibitor. Increased cyclic adenosine monophosphate (cAMP) interferes with platelet aggregation and mediates arterial vasodilation.

Pharmacokinetics: It undergoes CYP3A4 metabolism and excreted mainly in urine (74%). t½ is 11-13 hours. Peak pharmacodynamics effect occurs in 6 hours. For claudication 2-4 weeks is required for symptomatic relief.

Uses: Antiplatelet therapy for secondary prevention of noncardioembolic ischemic stroke or transient ischemic attack (TIA) and intermittent claudication.

Dose: 100 mg twice daily.

Adverse effects: Nausea, diarrhea, headache, peripheral edema, palpitation, and tachycardia.

Use in special population: Caution advised in moderate to severe hepatic impairment and severe renal failure. No safety data is available in pediatric population (below 18 years). It belongs to pregnancy category C. Discontinue nursing or drug during lactation. It is contraindicated in heart failure and hemostatic disorders.

CINNARIZINE

Introduction: Piperazine derivative with antihistaminic and antimuscarinic action.

Pharmacodynamics: It antagonizes histamine and has calcium channel-blocking property. It inhibits calcium translocation across the vestibular sensory cells in the ampullae and maintains endolymph flow by preventing constriction of the stria vascularis.

Pharmacokinetics: It is well absorbed from GI tract and peak plasma concentration is reached in 1–4 hours. Terminal t½ is 23 hours. It is metabolized by CYP2D6 in liver.

Uses: Treatment of vestibular disorders, motion sickness, and peripheral vascular disease (as it improves microcirculation).

Dose: 25 mg 2 hours before travel and then 12.5 mg every 8 hours duration of the journey for motion sickness. For Ménière's disease 25 mg three times day per oral is recommended. Cinnarizine is available in fixed dose combination with dimenhydrinate. This combination is favored for its dual mechanism of action. Dimenhydrinate inhibits central vestibular nuclei whereas cinnarizine inhibits peripheral labyrinth, thus effectively suppressing vertigo.

Adverse effects: Anticholinergic effects, drowsiness, weight gain, depression, acute dystonia, rarely parkinsonism, and tardive dyskinesia.

Use in special population: Dose reduction is needed in hepatic or renal failure. No adequate data regarding its use in pregnancy and lactation.

CITICOLINE

Introduction: Chemically it is cytidine-5'-diphosphocholine (CDP-choline). It is an important intermediate in the production of structural phospholipids of cell membranes. It is proposed to have neuroprotective effects.

Pharmacodynamics: After metabolism choline and cytidine are released. Choline is important in synthesis of acetyl choline, a vital neurotransmitter in brain. It inhibits phospholipase A2 activity thereby reducing free radical production, lowers glutamate concentration and increases phosphatidylcholine synthesis.

Pharmacokinetics: It has good oral bioavailability (>90%). Peak plasma concentration is reached in 1 hour. t½ is

50 hours for respiratory metabolism. It takes 70 hours for urinary excretion. It is excreted as carbon dioxide via respiration and some by urine.

Uses: Cognitive impairment, ischemic stroke, depression, schizophrenia, and glaucoma (clinical trial results have been inconsistent).

Dose: Oral and parenteral routes are available. 500–1,000 mg twice daily for 12 months.

Adverse effects: Abdominal pain and diarrhea.

Use in special population: No data is available in pregnancy, lactation, renal, and hepatic impairment.

CLADRIBINE

Introduction: Synthetic purine nucleoside used as an anticancer drug.

Pharmacodynamics: It is converted to cladribine triphosphate by deoxycytidine kinase intracellularly. This triphosphate form inhibits deoxyribonucleic acid (DNA) repair, synthesis, ATP depletion and apoptosis of lymphocytes.

Pharmacokinetics: t½ is 4–9 hours for IV form and eliminated by kidneys.

Uses: Hairy cell leukemias (first-line), chronic lymphocytic leukemia, cutaneous T cell lymphoma, and non-Hodgkin lymphoma. Oral form is the FDA approved for relapsing remitting multiple sclerosis.

Dose: 1.75 mg/kg/year. Treatment is given over 4–5 consecutive days in 1st and 2nd month. 12 months later second course starts as the same schedule given earlier.

Adverse effects: Opportunistic infections, lymphopenia, nausea, rash, fatigue, and pyrexia.

Use in special population: No specific dosage recommendation is available for its use in renal or liver failure. It is contraindicated in patients on other immunosuppressant, human immunodeficiency virus (HIV), tuberculosis, and pregnancy. Discontinue nursing or the drug regarding lactation.

CLOBAZAM

Introduction: It is the only benzodiazepine with nitrogen atoms at 1 and 5 position. All other benzodiazepines have nitrogen atom at 1 and 4 position. Has anxiolytic property too.

Pharmacodynamics: It binds to GABA-A receptor and increases the frequency of opening of chloride channels resulting in hyperpolarization and neuronal inhibition.

Pharmacokinetics: It is metabolized in liver by CYP3A4, and to a lesser extent by CYP2C19 and CYP2B6. N-desmethylclobazam is the active metabolite that is metabolized principally by CYP2C19. Peak plasma concentration in 0.5-4 hours. It has good oral bioavailability. t½ is 36-42 hours for clobazam and 71-82 hours for N-desmethylclobazam. Inactive metabolites are eliminated by renal excretion (82%). Genetic polymorphism of CYP2C19 influences pharmacokinetic and pharmacodynamic property of clobazam.

Uses: It is a broad-spectrum drug used as adjunctive therapy in focal, generalized, and myoclonic seizures. It is also FDA approved for Lennox–Gastaut syndrome in patients ≥2 years of age as an adjunctive therapy. It is used as a short term (2-4 weeks) therapy for anxiety.

Dose:
- *Children ≥2 years of age weighing ≤30 kg*: Start with 5 mg. In the next week 10 mg in two divided doses. Maximum dose is 20 mg/day.
- *Children ≥2 years of age weighing >30 kg*: Start with 10 mg. In the next week 20 mg in two divided doses. Maximum 40 mg/day.

Adverse effects: Sedation, abrupt withdrawal effect (may precipitate seizures), aggression, insomnia, irritability, ataxia, psychomotor hyperactivity, dysarthria, pyrexia, and fatigue.

Use in special population: It can cause profound sedation if given in patients on opioid or other benzodiazepine. In mild to moderate hepatic failure, half the recommended dose is given. In severe liver failure, data is insufficient. There is no need for dose reduction up to creatinine clearance (CrCl) of 30 mL/min. Use in pregnancy only if benefits outweigh risk. Monitor infants who are breastfed by mothers on clobazam.

CLOMIPRAMINE

Introduction: Tricyclic antidepressant.

Pharmacodynamics: Enhances norepinephrine and serotonin neurotransmission by inhibiting their reuptake into presynaptic terminal. It also blocks histamine receptor H1, alpha-1 adrenergic, and muscarinic receptor too.

Pharmacokinetics: t½ of parent drug and active metabolite are 32 and 69 hours. Oral bioavailability is 50%. Peak plasma concentration in 2-6 hours. Clinical response occurs between 2 and 6 weeks. Metabolized by CYP2D6, CYP1A2, and to a lesser extent by CYP3A4. Metabolites are excreted by kidneys.

Uses: Obsessive-compulsive disorder (OCD), chronic pain, panic disorder, major depression, cataplexy (symptomatic management), and eating disorders.

Dose: For OCD 25 mg to begin and raise to 100 mg in 2 weeks (maximum 250 mg). For children >10 years of age maximum dose is 100 mg/day. 100-250 mg for depression and chronic neuropathic pain. 25-200 mg for cataplexy.

Adverse effects: Anticholinergic side effects include dry mouth, constipation, and tachycardia. Sedation, weight gain and orthostatic hypotension, prolonged QT interval, increased suicidal tendency, and sexual dysfunction.

Use in special population: Belongs to category C. Discontinue nursing or drug. <10 years no safety data. Caution in liver and renal disease warranted.

CLONAZEPAM

Introduction: Benzodiazepine.

Pharmacodynamics: It binds to GABA-A receptor and increases the frequency of opening of chloride channels resulting in hyperpolarization and neuronal inhibition.

Pharmacokinetics: Peak plasma concentration is reached in 1-4 hours. Absolute bioavailability is approximately 90%. t½ is 18-50 hours. It undergoes CYP3A4 metabolism.

Uses: Myoclonic seizures, generalized tonic-clonic seizures, absence seizures refractory to ethosuximide, catatonia, akathisia, panic disorder, and refractory seizures.

Dose:
- *Infants and children <10 years of age or weighing <30 kg*: Initially, 0.01-0.03 mg/kg daily; initial dosage should not exceed 0.05 mg/kg daily given in two or three divided doses. Maintenance dosage of 0.1-0.2 mg/kg daily.
- *Children ≥10 years of age or weighing ≥30 kg*: Initial dosage should not exceed 1.5 mg daily given in three

divided doses. Increase dosage in increments of 0.5–1 mg every third day (up to a maximum dosage of 20 mg daily) until seizure control is achieved with minimal adverse effects.

Adverse effects: Sedation, drowsiness, ataxia, hypotonia, behavioral disturbances (principally in children) including aggressiveness, irritability, agitation, and hyperkinesis.

Use in special population: It belongs to pregnancy category D. Discontinue nursing or drug with respect to lactation. In hepatic impairment it is not advisable. Caution warranted in renal failure. Initiate at lower dose in elderly.

CLONIDINE

Introduction: It is an alpha-2 selective adrenergic receptor agonist.

Pharmacodynamics: By acting on CNS alpha-2 receptors it reduces the sympathetic outflow thereby decreasing blood pressure (BP). It also stimulates parasympathetic system and reduces heart rate. Norepinephrine, neuropeptide Y, and ATP release from postsympathetic nerve terminals are reduced when clonidine activates presynaptic alpha-2 receptors which also accounts for its antihypertensive effect.

Pharmacokinetics: It has a t½ of 6–24 hours and undergoes renal excretion. Oral bioavailability is 100%. Maximum plasma concentration is reached in 1–3 hours.

Uses: Though it is an antihypertensive drug it has many off-label uses in neurological disorders. ADHD, Tourette syndrome, hyperhidrosis, mania, postherpetic neuralgia, psychosis, and restless leg syndrome are some of the off-label uses where the drug has exhibited efficacy.

Dose: For tics and ADHD start at 0.05 mg at bedtime. Increase the dose by 0.05 mg every week to a maximum tolerable dose of 0.3 mg in three divided doses.

Adverse effects: Xerostomia and sedation are common side effects which may reduce in a few weeks of drug intake. Bradycardia and sexual dysfunction can occur. Transdermal patch can cause irritant dermatitis.

Use in special population: t½ (41 hours) increases in renal failure hence dose reduction is needed. It belongs to pregnancy category C and caution warranted during lactation.

CLOPIDOGREL

Introduction: Thienopyridines prodrug which inhibits P2Y12 receptors.

Pharmacodynamics: Platelet contains P2Y1 and P2Y12 receptors. Both receptors are G protein coupled proteins for ADP. ADP activated platelets receptor P2Y12 decreases intracellular cAMP which helps in platelet activation. Clopidogrel is an irreversible inhibitor of P2Y12 thereby preventing platelet activation. Slow onset and slow offset is because of its irreversible action on platelets.

Pharmacokinetics: Inhibition of platelet activation is seen 2 hours after ingestion of a loading dose of clopidogrel, and platelets are affected for the rest of their life span. First the drug undergoes hydrolysis and then thiol metabolite is formed by CYP isoenzymes (2C19, 2B6, and 1A2). Metabolic activation of clopidogrel needs CYP2C19 whose polymorphism can affect pharmacological effect of this drug. t½ is 6 hours for a single dose of 75 mg.

Uses: The FDA approved indications are to reduce the rate of stroke in TIAs, myocardial infarction, secondary prevention of ischemic stroke, peripheral artery disease, or acute coronary syndrome.

Dose: 300 mg loading and 75 mg is the maintenance dose.

Adverse effects: Thrombotic thrombocytopenic purpura (TTP) is rare. Bleeding risk is more particularly when combined with aspirin or anticoagulant.

Use in special population: Do not administer with proton pump inhibitors as they inhibit CYP2C19 which results in reduced conversion to active metabolite. No dose adjustment is needed in hepatic failure, renal failure, or geriatric population. It is contraindicated in active bleeding.

CLOZAPINE

Introduction: Dibenzodiazepine-derivative and atypical antipsychotic.

Pharmacodynamics: Antagonist activity at dopamine type 2 (D2) and serotonin type 2A (5-HT2A) receptors.

Pharmacokinetics: Bioavailability is 60% and reaches maximum plasma concentration in 2.5 hours. It undergoes liver metabolism by CYP1A2. Norclozapine is the major metabolite. t½ is 12 hours (4–66) with chronic dosing and t½ of norclozapine is 22.5 hours. Smoking 7–12 cigarettes per day induces CYP1A2 and reduces the drug levels. Fluvoxamine increase the drug 5- to 10-fold. CYP3A4 or 2D6 strong inhibitors increase the drug levels by twofold. CYP inducers also reduce the drug levels.

Uses: Treatment resistant schizophrenia and reduces suicide risk in schizophrenia and schizoaffective disorders.

Dose: Start with 12.5 mg once or twice daily. Increase 25 mg every 2 weeks till 300–400 mg is reached. Some patients may need 600–900 mg.

Adverse effects: Neutropenia (mechanism not known and not dose dependent), anticholinergic side effects, hypotension, syncope, tachycardia, sedation, headache, and tremor.

Use in special population: Dose reduction is needed in hepatic, renal impairment, and geriatric population. CYP2D6 poor metabolizers may require lower doses. Start therapy only when absolute neutrophil count is ≥1,500/mm^3. Monitor weekly neutrophil count every week for first 6 months, every 2 weeks for next 6 months, monthly thereafter.

COENZYME Q10

Introduction: Fat-soluble vitamin like molecule present in cell membrane. Also known as ubiquinone.

Pharmacodynamics: It is necessary for electron transfer in mitochondrial respiratory chain to produce ATP. It reduces lipid peroxidation and increase the production of antioxidant enzymes like superoxide dismutase. It is not FDA approved.

Pharmacokinetics: Peak plasma concentration is reached in 5–8 hours. It is metabolized in all tissues. Elimination is via biliary and fecal excretion.

Uses: Fibromyalgia, diabetes, cancer, heart failure, and neurodegenerative. Mitochondrial and muscular diseases are associated with decreased circulating levels of coenzyme Q10.

Dose: Oral supplements range from 30 to 600 mg/unit and are easily available over-the-counter.

Adverse effects: Stomach upset, nausea, vomiting, and diarrhea. Mild insomnia if dose is >100 mg/day.

Use in special population: It is not advised in biliary obstruction. Data in renal failure is not available. Coenzyme

Q supplements should be avoided in renal impairment. It is not advised in pregnancy and lactation.

CONIVAPTAN

Introduction: Nonselective (V1a receptor/V2 receptor) vasopressin antagonist.

Pharmacodynamics: It antagonizes vasopressin and causes free water excretion (aquaresis).

Pharmacokinetics: It is metabolized by CYP system in liver. t½ is 5–12 hours. It is highly protein bound and partially eliminated by kidney.

Uses: Only IV formulation is available and used in hypervolemic and euvolemic hyponatremia patients who are hospitalized (FDA approved).

Dose: Premixed injection containing 0.2 mg/mL of conivaptan hydrochloride in 5% dextrose injection is available. 20 mg loading in hypovolemic hyponatremia over 30 minutes followed by 20 mg IV continuous infusion over 24 hours for 2–4 days. Discontinue, if serum sodium rises >12 mEq/day, hypotension, or hypovolemia occurs.

Adverse effects: Headache, hyperglycemia, hypokalemia, polyuria, dizziness, dehydration, hypotension, xerostomia, and thirst.

Use in special population: It is contraindicated in hypovolemic hyponatremia, patients on CYP3A4 inhibitors, and anuria. Half the recommended dose is advised in mild to severe hepatic impairment and mild-to-moderate renal failure (30–60 mL/minute CrCl). In severe renal failure (<30 mL/minute), it is contraindicated. It belongs to pregnancy category C and breastfeeding is advised if benefits outweigh risk.

CYCLOPHOSPHAMIDE

Introduction: It is a nitrogen mustard.

Pharmacodynamics: It is an alkylating agent that prevents cell division by cross-linking DNA strands and decreasing DNA synthesis. It is a cell cycle phase nonspecific agent. It also possesses potent immunosuppressive activity.

Pharmacokinetics: It has a t½ of 3–12 hours (IV); children: 4 hours; adults: 6–8 hours. Its oral bioavailability is >75%. It undergoes hepatic metabolism to form its active metabolites acrolein, 4-aldophosphamide, 4-hydroperoxycyclophosphamide, and nor-nitrogen mustard. Its excretion is mainly in the urine.

Uses: Apart from oncological indications, it is used as a steroid sparing agent in myasthenia gravis, immune-mediated neuropathies, vasculitic neuropathy, and inflammatory myositis.

Dose: 1,000 mg/m^2 every 4 weeks × 6 months (NIH protocol) with pre- and postdrug hydration of 1–1.5 L is recommended.

Adverse effects: Common adverse side effects reported in several studies and clinical trials include hemorrhagic cystitis (prevented by administration of mesna), amenorrhea, myelosuppression, alopecia, and spells of nausea and vomiting.

Use in special population: No dosage adjustment in renal disease with CrCl > 30 mL/min. 50–75% of the dose is given in patients with CrCl < 30 mL/min. It crosses the placenta and is teratogenic. It is not recommended for use in breastfeeding mothers as the drug and its metabolites have been detected in breast milk.

CYCLOSPORINE

Introduction: Calcineurin inhibitor and immunosuppressant.

Pharmacodynamics: Inhibition of lymphocytic proliferation and function.

Pharmacokinetics: It is metabolized by CYP3A4. Peak blood and plasma concentrations are attained about 3.5 hours following oral administration. Terminal t½ is 8.4–27 hours. 6% is excreted in urine, whereas majority is excreted in bile.

Uses: Used as a steroid-sparing agent in myasthenia gravis, immune-mediated neuropathies, and inflammatory myositis. Organ transplant recipients receive to prevent rejection in combination with other immunosuppressants.

Dose: Start 100 mg twice daily. Maintenance dose is 3–6 mg/kg/day, divided in two daily doses.

Adverse effects: Posterior reversible encephalopathy syndrome (PRES), tremor, seizures, nephrotoxicity, hypertension, infection, hepatotoxicity, hirsutism, tremor, gum hyperplasia, and neoplasia.

Use in special population: Monitor CBC, LFT, renal function test (RFT), and BP. It belongs to pregnancy category C. Breastfeeding is not recommended.

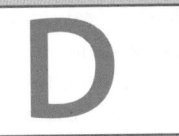

Section Outline

- Dabigatran
- Dalfampridine
- Dantrolene
- Darifenacin
- Deflazacort
- Delandistrogene moxeparvovec
- Desipramine
- Dexamethasone
- Diazepam
- Dihydroergotamine
- Dimenhydrinate
- Dimethyl fumarate
- Dipyridamole
- Donepezil
- Dosulepin
- Doxepin
- Droxidopa (L-Threo-3,4,-Dihydroxyphenylserine)
- Duloxetine

DABIGATRAN

Introduction: It is an oral direct thrombin inhibitor and synthetically derived.

Pharmacodynamics: Dabigatran etexilate is a prodrug that gets converted to dabigatran by esterases and binds to thrombin that is circulating free as well as clot bound. It blocks thrombin in a competitive and reversible manner. Ultimately thrombin-mediated conversion of fibrinogen to fibrin is inhibited.

Pharmacokinetics: It has a poor oral bioavailability of about 6% and a half-life ($t\frac{1}{2}$) of 12–14 hours. Plasma concentration peaks in 2 hours. About 80% of the drug is eliminated unchanged by kidneys. Drug should be swallowed as a whole and not chewed. Anticoagulation monitoring is not necessary. It is substrate for P-glycoprotein, hence drug like rifampicin lower the drug concentration whereas drugs such as ketoconazole and verapamil increase the drug levels.

Uses: Venous thromboembolism, stroke prevention in nonvalvular atrial fibrillation, and thromboprophylaxis in hip and knee surgeries.

Dose: 150 mg twice daily capsules.

Adverse effects: Bleeding, concomitant use with nonsteroidal anti-inflammatory drugs (NSAIDs) and antiplatelets increase the risk of bleeding. Annual bleeding risk is same as that of warfarin (3%). Intracranial bleed is 70% lesser than warfarin but gastrointestinal (GI) bleeding rate is higher (particularly in people aged above 75 years). Idarucizumab is reversal agent for dabigatran and can be used in life-threatening bleed.

Use in special population: Half the usual dose is advised in severe renal failure [15–30 mL/min creatinine clearance (CrCl)]. It is contraindicated in triple-positive antiphospholipid antibody syndrome (positive for lupus anticoagulant, anticardiolipin antibodies, and anti–β2-glycoprotein I antibodies) and in patients with prothetic valves. No data regarding its use in pregnancy and lactation. Efficacy and safety established for pediatric (3 months to 18 years) usage in venous thromboembolism.

DALFAMPRIDINE

Introduction: A potassium channel blocker previously known as 4-aminopyridine.

Pharmacodynamics: It is a broad-spectrum potassium channel blocker and result in improvement in conduction of action potential in demyelinated axons. This clinically translates to improvement in walking.

Pharmacokinetics: Though metabolized by CYP2E1, majority of the drug is eliminated by kidneys unchanged. t½ is 5–6 hours. Oral bioavailability is 96% for extended release form.

Uses: Improves gait in multiple sclerosis patients.

Dose: 10 mg twice daily.

Adverse effects: Insomnia, dizziness, headache, nausea, malaise, and back ache.

Use in special population: It is contraindicated in patients with seizures and renal failure (CrCl < 50 mL/min). No manufacturer recommendation is available for its use in hepatic impairment. No adequate data is available regarding its use in pregnancy and lactation.

DANTROLENE

Introduction: Skeletal muscle relaxant.

Pharmacodynamics: It blocks the ryanodine receptors within the sarcoplasmic reticulum, which inhibits the release of calcium ions necessary for the contraction process to occur.

Pharmacokinetics: It undergoes liver metabolism to form 5-hydroxydantrolene and an acetyl amino metabolite. Further metabolism involves hydrolysis and oxidation to form nitrophenylfuroic acid. Urine and bile excretion is the route of elimination. t½ for intravenous (IV) route is 4–11.4 hours whereas it is 9 hours following oral administration.

Uses: Malignant hyperthermia [IV formulation labeled as orphan drug by the Food and Drug Administration (FDA)], spasticity, and off-label use in neuroleptic malignant syndrome.

Dose: Oral dose in adults is 25 mg once daily for 7 days, followed by 25 mg three times daily for 7 days, then 50 mg three times daily for 7 days, and then 100 mg three times daily, if necessary. For treatment of malignant hyperthermia 1 mg/kg or more by rapid IV injection. Maximum total dose is of 10 mg/kg.

Adverse effects: Drowsiness, fatigue, nausea, muscle weakness, dizziness, and dyspnea.

Use in special population: Prior liver function test (LFT) and periodic LFT monitoring is needed. It is contraindicated in active liver disease. It belongs to pregnancy category C. Discontinue nursing or drug during lactation based on the situation.

DARIFENACIN

Introduction: It is selective M3 muscarinic receptor antagonist.

Pharmacodynamics: M3 receptor blockade results in inhibition of acetylcholine release from postganglionic parasympathetic nerve endings, thereby increasing bladder capacity, lowering intravesical pressure and reducing the frequency of bladder contractions.

Pharmacokinetics: It undergoes hepatic metabolism and by CYP2D6 and CYP3A4. It has a short t½ of 3–4 hours in immediate release oral form, hence prolonged release is preferred (14–16 hours).

Uses: Overactive bladder.

Dose: 7.5 and 15 mg prolonged release form once daily.

Adverse effects: Dry mouth, abdominal discomfort, constipation, and blurred vision. Confusion and delirium are less as it has got M3 selectivity and spares M1 receptor which are in abundance in central nervous system (CNS).

Use in special population: There are no studies in pregnant women. Dose reduction needed in liver dysfunction and if used along with drugs that inhibit CYP2D6 and CYP3A4.

DEFLAZACORT

Introduction: Deflazacort is a corticosteroid prodrug slightly less potent than prednisone. Unwanted side effects of steroids particularly regarding bone metabolism and hyperglycemia are lesser with deflazacort. But this data was from small and short duration trials. 6 mg of deflazacort is equal to 5 mg of prednisone.

Pharmacodynamics: It is converted to active metabolite namely 21-desDFZ and acts through the glucocorticoid receptor to exert anti-inflammatory and immunosuppressive effects. The exact mechanism by which deflazacort exerts its therapeutic effects in patients with Duchenne muscular dystrophy (DMD) is not known.

Pharmacokinetics: Median time to peak plasma concentration is about 1 hour. Oral bioavailability is 70%. Principally drug is eliminated by renal (about 68%) excretion. 21-desDFZ is metabolized by CYP3A4. t½ is 1.5–2 hours.

Uses: FDA approved in children aged ≥5 years with DMD to improve muscle function and strength.

Dose: 0.9 mg/kg daily. Reduce the dose to one-third if used with CYP inhibitors.

Adverse effects: Mood and behavior disturbance, adrenocortical insufficiency on withdrawal, hypokalemia, salt and water retention, hyperglycemia, Cushing syndrome, infections such as herpes simplex virus (HSV) and varicella-zoster virus (VZV), decreased bone mineral density, avascular necrosis, myopathy, serious skin rashes, cataract, and bruising.

Use in special population: No dose reduction is needed in mild to moderate hepatic impairment. No adjustment is needed for severe renal disease. Use in pregnancy only if benefits outweigh risk. Monitor newborn baby as it is distributed in breast milk and nursing should be continued when benefits of breastfeeding outweigh risk.

DELANDISTROGENE MOXEPARVOVEC

Introduction: Gene therapy using adeno-associated virus as a vector. First gene therapy approved to treat DMD.

Pharmacodynamics: Three parts namely vector, promoter, and transgene. Vector here used in AAVrh74 serotype that has affinity for skeletal and cardiac muscle. The promoter MHCK7 enhances the transgene expression. Transgene encodes a microdystrophin protein consisting of selected domains of dystrophin expressed in normal muscle cells.

Pharmacokinetics: Data not available.

Uses: Ambulatory patients ≥4 years of age with DMD who have a confirmed mutation in the *DMD* gene. Can be used in nonambulatory patients also.

Dose: Available strength 1.33×10^{13} vector genomes (vg)/mL 10 mL vials. In patients 10–70 kg, 1.33×10^{14} vg/kg of body weight. Infusion over 1–2 hours.

Adverse effects: Infusion-related reactions including hypersensitivity and anaphylaxis, hepatitis, myocarditis, and myositis. Common adverse effects include vomiting and nausea, pyrexia, and thrombocytopenia.

Use in special population: While handling patient waste, caution advised at least for a month after infusion as virus shedding occurs through body waste. Corticosteroids may be required before and after infusion. Administration is not recommended in patients with elevated anti-AAVrh74 total binding antibody titers (≥1:400) and exon 8 and exon 9 deletion in *DMD* gene. It is contraindicated in pregnancy and lactation. No data is available regarding its use in liver and renal impairment.

DESIPRAMINE

Introduction: Secondary amine; belongs to tricyclic antidepressant.

Pharmacodynamics: It enhances norepinephrine and serotonin neurotransmission by inhibiting their reuptake into presynaptic terminal. It also blocks histamine receptor H1, alpha 1 adrenergic, and muscarinic receptor too.

Pharmacokinetics: It undergoes liver metabolism by CYP2D6, 1A2, and 2C. Urine excretion of metabolites is around 70%. t½ is 7 to >60 hours. Peak plasma levels are achieved in 4–6 hours. Antidepressant effect takes 3 weeks.

Uses: FDA approved for depression. Off-label use for bulimia nervosa, irritable bowel syndrome, neuropathic pain, overactive bladder, postherpetic neuralgia, and attention deficit hyperactivity disorder.

Dose: Available in 10 and 25 mg. Start at 25–50 mg/day. Increase up to 100–200 mg/day. Maximum dose is 300 mg/day.

Adverse effects: Withdrawal effects (flu-like syndrome), anticholinergic side effects include dry mouth, constipation, tachycardia, sedation, weight gain and orthostatic hypotension, prolonged QT interval, increased suicidal tendency, and sexual dysfunction.

Use in special population: It belongs to pregnancy category C and in lactation drug is not recommended. In children <12 years, safety is not established. Avoid in geriatric age >65 years. No specific guidance given for its usage in renal and liver failure. It is contraindicated in patients who had monoamine oxidase inhibitor (MAOI) in last 14 days and recovering phase of myocardial infarction.

DEXAMETHASONE

Introduction: Synthetic glucocorticoid with minimal mineralocorticoid activity.

Pharmacodynamics: Similar to deflazacort.

Pharmacokinetics: Duration of anti-inflammatory action lasts 2.75 days for a 5 mg dose. It is metabolized in liver by CYP3A4 system.

Uses: Bacterial and tuberculous meningitis, cerebral edema, and metastatic spinal cord compression.

Dose:
- In bacterial meningitis—0.15 mg/kg four times daily for the first 2–4 days of anti-infective therapy has been administered.
- In tuberculous meningitis—0.4 mg/kg/day IV in 1st week, 0.3 mg/kg/day IV in 2nd week, 0.2 mg/kg/day IV in 3rd week, 0.1 mg/kg/day IV in 4th week. Following IV regimen oral dexamethasone is started at 4 mg/day for the 5th week. Each week 1 mg is tapered and stopped.
- In cerebral edema—initially, 10 mg IV, then 4 mg IM every 6 hours for 2–4 days, then taper over 5–7 days.
- In metastatic spinal cord compression—IV or oral dexamethasone is given at a dose of 16 mg/day.

Adverse effects: Similar to deflazacort.

Use in special population: Liver cirrhosis patients exhibit exaggerated glucocorticoid response. Use with caution in renal impairment. Gradually withdraw systemic glucocorticoids until recovery of hypothalamic–pituitary–adrenal (HPA) axis function occurs following long-term therapy with pharmacologic dosages.

DIAZEPAM

Introduction: Benzodiazepine, anticonvulsant, anxiolytic, sedative, and skeletal muscle relaxant.

Pharmacodynamics: It binds to GABAA receptor and increases the frequency of opening of chloride channels resulting in hyperpolarization and neuronal inhibition.

Pharmacokinetics: Metabolized by CYP2C19 and CYP3A4 and excreted in urine. Intramuscular (IM) absorption is erratic. Oral and rectal has good bioavailability. Onset of action via IV route is in 1–5 minutes. Duration of effect lasts 15–60 minutes. t½ of diazepam is 20–50 hours.

Metabolites of diazepam and their t½: Desmethyldiazepam 30–200 hours, temazepam 5–20 hours, and oxazepam 3–21 hours.

Uses: Anxiety, alcohol withdrawal, status epilepticus, spasticity, and sedation.

Dose: IM, IV, oral, and rectal formulations available.
- For anxiety and spasticity in adults—oral dose 2–10 mg two to four times daily, depending on severity of symptoms.
- For alcohol withdrawal—10 mg three or four times during the first 24 hours, followed by 5 mg three or four times daily as needed.

For seizure:
- Oral 2–10 mg two to four times daily for adjunctive management of seizure disorders.
- 0.2 mg/kg as rectal gel.
- IV initially, 5–10 mg. May repeat at 10–15-minute intervals, if necessary, up to a maximum total dose of 30 mg.
- In children >5 years for seizures 1 mg IV. May repeat in 2–5 minutes to a maximum dose of 10 mg.
- Rectal gel in 2–5 years 0.5 mg/kg.
- In >5 years 0.3 mg/kg.

Adverse effects: Drowsiness, ataxia, muscle weakness, fatigue, respiratory depression, and withdrawal seizures.

Use in special population: Dose reduction is needed in hepatic and renal involvement to avoid oversedation. Concomitant administration with opioid is avoided. Belongs to pregnancy category D. Avoid nursing or drug with respect to lactation. In geriatric population, begin with lower doses.

DIHYDROERGOTAMINE

Introduction: Ergot alkaloid.

Pharmacodynamics: 5-HT1B/1D agonist and cause selective vasoconstriction.

Pharmacokinetics: It is metabolized by CYP3A4 system in liver and it is also a CYP3A inhibitor. It undergoes high first pass metabolism, hence poor oral bioavailability. Action starts in 5, 15 and 30 minutes following IV, IM, and subcutaneous respectively. t½ is 9 hours.

Uses: Acute treatment of migraine and cluster headache, IV form in status migrainosus. It is not used in basilar or hemiplegic migraine and also not used as a prophylaxis.

Dose:
- Oral, IV, IM, subcutaneous, and nasal formulation available.
- 0.5 mg in each nostril—nasal formulation
- 1 mg direct IV or IM or subcutaneous followed by 1 mg after 1 hour if attack persists.
- Maximum 2 mg in 24 hours if IV otherwise maximum 3 mg. Total week dose is 6 mg maximum.

Adverse effects: Paresthesia, hypertension, flushing, anxiety, and diarrhea. Intranasal form cause rhinitis and taste disturbance.

Use in special population: It is contraindicated in pregnancy (category X), lactation, ischemic heart disease, concomitant triptan usage, peripheral arterial disease, severe liver or renal failure, basilar, or hemiplegic migraine.

DIMENHYDRINATE

Introduction: Ethanolamine-derivative antihistamine containing a diphenhydramine moiety; antiemetic.

Pharmacodynamics: Antihistaminic, CNS depressant, antiemetic, and anticholinergic activity contribute to the therapeutic effect. It inhibits vestibular stimulation arising from otolith and semicircular canals.

Pharmacokinetics: It is metabolized in liver and excreted by kidneys. It is an orally well-absorbed drug. Therapeutic effect lasts 3–6 hours.

Uses: Motion sickness, symptomatic management of vertigo, nausea, vomiting in Ménière's disease and other vestibular disorders.

Dose: Oral, IM, and IV forms are available. For prevention of motion sickness start 50–100 mg 30 minutes prior to journey. Repeat every 4–6 hours and do not exceed 400 mg/day. For acute attack of Ménière's disease 50 mg IM can be given. 25–50 mg thrice daily for maintenance of symptom relief in Ménière's disease.

Adverse effects: Dry mouth, palpitations, orthostatic hypotension, incoordination, drowsiness, headache, and blurred vision.

Use in special population: No specific recommendation is available for its use in renal and hepatic impairment. It belongs to pregnancy category C. Discontinue nursing or the drug during lactation period. Safety not established in children below 2 years.

DIMETHYL FUMARATE

Introduction: Fumaric acid derivative with immuno-modulatory activity and used as a disease-modifying agent in multiple sclerosis.

Pharmacodynamics: Exact mechanism of action is not known. Nuclear factor (erythroid-derived 2)-like 2 (Nrf2) is activated by dimethyl fumarate (DMF) and monomethyl fumarate (MMF). This action may result in inhibition of lymphocyte proliferation and hematopoietic stem cells.

Pharmacokinetics: MMF is the active form formed by esterases acting on DMF. Peak plasma concentration occurs in 2–2.5 hours. MMF enters Krebs cycle. 60% of the drug is eliminated by CO_2 exhalation. Its t½ is 1 hour.

Uses: Clinically isolated syndrome (CIS), relapsing-remitting multiple sclerosis (RRMS), and secondary progressive multiple sclerosis (SPMS).

Dose: 120 mg twice daily after a week then 240 mg twice daily maintenance.

Adverse effects: Cutaneous flushing (nicotinic effect), lymphopenia, opportunistic infections and progressive multifocal leukoencephalopathy, liver injury, and rarely serious GI problems such as perforation and bleeding occurs.

Use in special population: LFT and complete blood count (CBC) to be monitored prior to initiation and periodically in patients on DMF. No dosage reduction is needed in hepatic, renal impairment, and geriatric population.

DIPYRIDAMOLE

Introduction: Antiplatelet agent and coronary vasodilator.

Pharmacodynamics: It inhibits phosphodiesterase and blocks uptake of adenosine. Adenosine activates platelet adenylyl cyclase and increases cyclic adenosine monophosphate (AMP) which interferes with platelet function.

Pharmacokinetics: Oral bioavailability (for combination form with aspirin) is 37–66%. Peak plasma concentration occurs in 45–150 minutes for conventional tablet and in 2 hours for combination form. It is metabolized in liver to monoglucuronide and eliminated in feces. Terminal t½ is 10–12 hours for conventional tablet and 13.6 hours for fixed combination.

Uses: An adjunct to coumarin anticoagulants in heart valve replacement, fixed dose combination of aspirin with dipyridamole secondary prevention of stroke who had transient ischemic attack (TIA) and history of thrombotic stroke. IV form is used as an adjunct to thallium-based myocardial perfusion imaging in patients unable to exercise adequately.

Dose: Conventional tablets (75–100 mg) four times a day. 200 mg of extended-release dipyridamole and 25 mg of aspirin (one capsule) twice daily in the morning and evening. If headache is not tolerable use at night alone and in morning use low-dose aspirin, resume twice daily dose within a week.

Adverse effects: GI intolerance, flushing, headache, dizziness, and rash. It may precipitate chest pain in coronary artery disease and can cause liver dysfunction.

Use in special population: It belongs to pregnancy category B for conventional tablet and category D for aspirin combination. Caution while breastfeeding. In children <12 years, safety is not established.

DONEPEZIL

Introduction: Reversible cholinesterase inhibitor.

Pharmacodynamics: By reversibly inhibiting acetylcholinesterase it prevents acetylcholine hydrolysis, thereby increases the availability of acetylcholine at the synapses (enhancing cholinergic transmission).

Pharmacokinetics: It has oral bioavailability of 100%. The drug reaches a peak plasma concentration within 3–4 hours.

CYP2D6, CYP3A4, and glucuronidation are the three major pathways of metabolism. It has prolonged t½ of 70 hours. Metabolites are excreted in urine.

Uses: Symptomatic treatment of mild or moderate dementia due to Alzheimer's disease (AD). Effect is generally modest, usually producing a 6- to 12-month delay in progression. Off-label use in traumatic brain injury, Lewy body dementia, Parkinson disease dementia, and vascular dementia.

Dose: Start at 5 mg initially, if tolerated increase up to 10 mg. It is also available in combination with memantine.

Adverse effects: Muscle cramps, abnormal dreams, and GI distress.

Use in special population: Caution is advised in patients with syncope or bradycardia (has vagotonic properties). It belongs to pregnancy category C and caution warranted during breastfeeding. No dose adjustment is required in renal or hepatic impairment.

DOSULEPIN

Introduction: Dosulepin is a thiol derivative of amitriptyline and has action and side effects similar to amitriptyline.

Pharmacodynamics: similar to other tricyclic antiepressants like amitriptyline.

Pharmacokinetics: Maximum plasma concentration reaches in 2 hours after an oral dose of 25 mg. The metabolic pathways of dosulepin involve N-demethylation, S-oxidation, and glucuronic acid conjugation. Metabolites are excreted in urine and its t½ is 20 hours.

Uses: Similar to amitriptyline.

Dose: Available in 25, 50, and 75 mg capsules. Begin with 25 mg at night. Gradually increase up to 75–150 mg based on clinical response. Maximum dose is 225 mg for depression and 150 mg for migraine.

Adverse effects: Similar to amitriptyline.

Use in special population: Similar to amitriptyline.

DOXEPIN

Introduction: Belongs to tricyclic antidepressant.

Pharmacodynamics: It enhances norepinephrine and serotonin neurotransmission by inhibiting their reuptake into presynaptic terminal. It also blocks histamine receptor H1, alpha-1 adrenergic, and muscarinic receptor too.

Pharmacokinetics: It is metabolized by CYP2D6, CYP1A2, and to a lesser extent by CYP3A4. Metabolites are excreted in urine. Terminal t½ is 15 hours for the parent drug and 31 hours for the metabolite nordoxepin.

Uses: FDA approved for major depressive disorder, anxiety, insomnia, and pruritus. It is used as an off-label treatment for neuropathic pain and migraine.

Dose: Topical doxepin (5%) is used in atopic dermatitis or lichen simplex chronicus. It is available as 10 and 25 mg capsules. Start at 25–75 mg at bedtime. Target dose is 100–300 mg. Increase the dose by every 3rd day.

Adverse effects: Anticholinergic side effects include dry mouth, constipation, tachycardia, sedation, weight gain, and orthostatic hypotension, prolonged QT interval, increased suicidal tendency, and sexual dysfunction.

Use in special population: It belongs to pregnancy category C and in lactation drug is not recommended. In children <12 years, safety is not established. Avoid in geriatric age >65 years. No specific guidance given for its usage in renal and liver failure. It is contraindicated in patients who had MAOI in last 14 days and recovering phase of myocardial infarction.

DROXIDOPA (L-THREO-3,4,-DIHYDROXYPHENYLSERINE)

Introduction: Droxidopa is a synthetic prodrug of norepinephrine.

Pharmacodynamics: It is converted by L-aromatic amino acid decarboxylase into norepinephrine.

Pharmacokinetics: It is metabolized by catecholamine pathway by enzymes such as catechol-O-methyltransferase (COMT) and DOPA decarboxylase. Metabolism do not involve CYP enzymes. Plasma concentration peaks in 1–4 hours and t½ is 2.5 hours.

Uses: Symptomatic neurogenic orthostatic hypotension in patients with primary autonomic failure, dopamine β-hydroxylase deficiency, or nondiabetic autonomic neuropathy. It is designated as an orphan drug by the FDA.

Dose: Initially taken at 100 mg three times day with or without food orally. Maximum doses is 1,800 mg in three divided doses. Efficacy beyond 2 weeks is not established and may need to reassess.

Adverse effects: Headache, nausea, vomiting, and supine hypertension are the common side effects. Avoid in heart failure, arrhythmias, and ischemic heart disease. Cases of neuroleptic malignant syndrome have been reported.

Use in special population: It belongs to pregnancy category C. Secretion into human breast milk is not known. No dose reduction is needed in mild to moderate renal failure.

DULOXETINE

Introduction: Serotonin-norepinephrine reuptake inhibitors (SNRIs); used as anxiolytic and antidepressant.

Pharmacodynamics: It inhibits reuptake of both serotonin and norepinephrine. Dopamine increases in prefrontal cortex as a result of reuptake inhibition. Serotonin and norepinephrine increases in descending spinal pathway on dorsal horn. It lacks antihistamine, antiadrenergic, and anticholinergic activity.

Pharmacokinetics: It undergoes CYP1A2 and CYP2D6 metabolism. Peak plasma concentration is attained in 6 hours. $t_{1/2}$ is 12 hours. Urine excretion of metabolites constitutes 70%.

Uses: Generalized anxiety disorder, neuropathic pain, fibromyalgia, stress urinary incontinence, and major depression.

Dose: Start at 30 mg. After a week increase up to 60 mg. Maintenance is 40–60 mg/day.

Adverse effects: Common adverse effects include diarrhea, decreased appetite, vomiting, hyperhidrosis, somnolence, insomnia, decreased libido, and sexual dysfunction. Serotonin syndrome risk if used with other SNRI, selective serotonin reuptake inhibitor (SSRI), triptan, and MAOI. Hyponatremia, transaminitis, and hepatic failure are some rare side effects.

Use in special population: In patients with CrCl of 30–80 mL/min lower initial dose. If CrCl is <30 mL/min, drug is not advisable. It belongs to pregnancy category C and lactation is not advised. In children <18 years, no safety is established. It is also not advised in hepatic impairment or concomitant alcohol ingestion (hepatotoxicity).

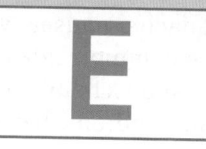

Section Outline

- Eculizumab
- Edaravone
- Efgartigimod alfa
- Eletriptan
- Entacapone
- Eptinezumab
- Erenumab
- Escitalopram
- Eslicarbazepine acetate
- Eteplirsen
- Ethosuximide
- Etizolam
- Ezogabine

ECULIZUMAB

Introduction: It is an immunoglobulin G (IgG) recombinant humanized monoclonal antibody against terminal complement.

Pharmacodynamics: It prevents the activation of terminal complement by binding to the C5 complement protein. This shields the neuromuscular junction from the damaging effects of antibody-mediated complement activation.

Pharmacokinetics: Its half-life (t½) is 270–375 hours. Metabolism of the drug is not well characterized. It takes 2 weeks to inhibit complement following a single dose.

Uses: Atypical hemolytic uremic syndrome and paroxysmal nocturnal hemoglobinuria are the hematological indications. In neurology, it is used as steroid-sparing immunosuppression agent in refractory generalized acetylcholine receptor (AChR) antibody positive myasthenia gravis. In neuromyelitis optica spectrum disorder (NMOSD), it is used to prevent relapses.

Dose: For patients with generalized myasthenia gravis, 900 mg intravenous (IV) weekly for the first 4 weeks, followed by 1,200 mg IV for the fifth dose 1 week later, then 1,200 mg IV every 2 weeks thereafter. For NMOSD 900 mg IV weekly for the first four doses, then 1,200 mg IV every 2 weeks. Given as IV over a period of 35 minutes and monitor for 1 hour postinfusion.

Adverse effects: Influenza-like illness, myalgia, nasopharyngitis, cough, headache, fatigue, and back pain. Serious, sometimes life-threatening or fatal meningococcal infections (e.g., sepsis and meningitis) have been reported.

Use in special population: Patients should receive meningococcal vaccine at least 2 weeks prior to first dose of eculizumab. It is contraindicated in active, severe *Neisseria meningitidis* infection. It belongs to pregnancy category C and caution warranted during lactation.

EDARAVONE

Introduction: It is a free radical scavenger used in amyotrophic lateral sclerosis (ALS). It is designated as an orphan drug by the Food and Drug Administration (FDA). It slows decline in functioning of the patient including motor, bulbar, and respiratory functions.

Pharmacodynamics: Exact mechanism of action is not known. Antioxidant property of the drug may help.

Pharmacokinetics: Metabolized by multiple uridine diphosphate-glucuronosyltransferase (UGT) enzymes. t½ is 4.5–9 hours. 60–80% of the drug is excreted in urine as glucuronide conjugates. 60 mg IV formulation is equal to 105 mg oral suspension. It reaches peak plasma concentration in 60 minutes IV and 30 minutes via oral route in fasting condition.

Uses: ALS and neuroprotective agent in ischemic stroke.

Dose: Oral suspension and IV forms are available. 60 mg is given as two consecutive 30 mg infusion over 1 hour. First cycle is 1–14 days IV therapy and next 14 days drug-free period. In subsequent cycles 10 doses out of first 14 days are administered followed by 14 day drug-free period. Same schedule to be followed for oral suspension except the dose is 105 mg.

Adverse effects: Gait disturbance, headache, and contusion.

Use in special population: Dosage adjustment not needed in liver failure and mild to moderate renal impairment. No data regarding its use in severe renal impairment. No adequate data regarding its use in pregnancy and lactation.

EFGARTIGIMOD ALFA

Introduction: It is a neonatal Fc receptor blocker; an immunomodulatory agent.

Pharmacodynamics: Human IgG1 antibody fragment binds to the neonatal Fc receptor (FcRn), resulting in the reduction of circulating IgG (pathogenic antibodies). This translates to clinical improvement in myasthenia patients.

Pharmacokinetics: t½ is 3–5 days. It undergoes degradation via proteolytic enzymes into small peptides and amino acids.

Uses: Generalized myasthenia gravis in adults who are anti-AChR antibody positive; generally as a third-line agent.

Dose: It is available as a 20 mg/mL (400 mg) single-dose vial. 10 mg/kg given as an IV infusion over 1 hour once weekly for 4 weeks. In adults weighing ≥120 kg, the recommended dosage is 1,200 mg (three vials) per infusion.

Adverse effects: Urinary tract infection, respiratory tract infection, headache, and infusion-related reactions.

Use in special population: No dose reduction recommended in hepatic or renal failure. No adequate studies in pregnancy and lactation. Breastfeeding can be continued and infant to be monitored. Safety not established in children.

ELETRIPTAN

Discussed under triptans.

ENTACAPONE

Introduction: It is a peripheral catechol-O-methyltransferase (COMT) inhibitor.

Pharmacodynamics: COMT inhibitors block the peripheral conversion of *levodopa* to 3-O-methyldopa, increasing both the plasma t½ of *levodopa* and the fraction of each dose that reaches the central nervous system (CNS).

Pharmacokinetics: It has short t½ of 2 hours. Oral bioavailability is 35% and peak plasma concentration is attained in 1 hour. Undergoes isomerization followed by glucuronidation to form inactive metabolite and 90% excreted in feces via bile.

Uses: Reduce significantly "wearing-off" symptoms in patients treated with *levodopa/carbidopa*.

Dose: 200 mg with each dose of levodopa, fixed dose with levodopa/carbidopa are also available. Maximum dose is 1.6 g/day.

Adverse effects: Nausea, orthostatic hypotension, vivid dreams, confusion, and hallucinations. No hepatotoxicity unlike tolcapone.

Use in special population: Use in pregnancy only if benefits outweigh risk. Caution warranted in lactating mothers on entacapone. No dose adjustment required in renal failure. Caution required when using in liver disease as biliary excretion is the major route of elimination.

EPTINEZUMAB

Introduction: It is a recombinant humanized IgG1 monoclonal antibody specific for calcitonin gene-related peptide (CGRP) ligand.

Pharmacodynamics: CGRP has a role in multiple pathophysiologic mechanisms underlying migraine attacks. It binds to alpha and beta isoforms of human CGRP and prevents activation of receptor. CGRP is a neuropeptide released in trigeminocervical complex system that plays a major role in cerebral vessels vasodilation and pain modulation.

Pharmacokinetics: It takes 4.8 hours to reach maximum plasma concentration. t½ is 27 days. It undergoes probable proteolytic degradation into small peptides.

Uses: Migraine prevention.

Dose: IV formulation 100 or 300 mg 3 months once IV.

Adverse effects: Constipation and injection site reaction.

Use in special population: No adequate data regarding its use in pregnancy. 5 months washout period required for pregnancy if on this monoclonal antibody. Pediatric safety is not established. No specific recommendations in renal or hepatic failure. Data on effect of this drug on lactation is inadequate.

ERENUMAB

Introduction: It is a recombinant humanized IgG2 monoclonal antibody specific for CGRP ligand.

Pharmacodynamics: It potently and competitively inhibits the binding of CGRP to its receptor. Other CGRP monoclonal antibodies target ligand. CGRP has a role in multiple pathophysiologic mechanisms underlying migraine attacks.

CGRP is a neuropeptide released in trigeminocervical complex system that plays a major role in cerebral vessels vasodilation and pain modulation.

Pharmacokinetics: It takes 6 days to reach maximum plasma concentration. t½ is 28 days. Undergoes probable proteolytic degradation into small peptides.

Uses: Migraine prophylaxis.

Dose: Subcutaneous (SC) 70 mg or 140 mg monthly.

Adverse effects: Constipation and injection site reaction. Monitor for new-onset or worsening hypertension.

Use in special population: No adequate data is available regarding its use in pregnancy. 5 months washout period required for pregnancy if on this monoclonal antibody. Pediatric safety is not established. No specific recommendations in renal or hepatic failure. Data regarding its use in lactating mothers is inadequate.

ESCITALOPRAM

Introduction: It belongs to selective serotonin reuptake inhibitors (SSRIs) and is S-enantiomer of citalopram.

Pharmacodynamics: Serotonin transporter (SERT) is responsible for the reuptake and clearance of 5HT in the brain. SSRI inhibits SERT resulting in increases serotonin availability in CNS.

Pharmacokinetics: It is metabolized in liver by CYP2C19 and CYP3A4 making them vulnerable for drug interactions. Elimination is by excretion in urine. Peak plasma concentration is reached in 5 hours. Orally well-absorbed.

Uses: Panic disorder, obsessive–compulsive disorder (OCD), generalized anxiety disorder, FDA approved for acute and maintenance treatment of major depressive disorder.

Dose: 10 mg/day. Can increase up to 20 mg/day after 1 week. 1–4 weeks needed for antidepressant effect.

Adverse effects: Insomnia, decreased libido, hyponatremia [syndrome of inappropriate antidiuretic hormone (SIADH)], sexual dysfunction (ejaculatory delay), hyperhidrosis, and fatigue are common adverse effects. QT prolongation and risk of suicidal tendency in first few weeks are possible. Abrupt withdrawal can cause dysphoric mood, headache, confusion, and anxiety. Risk of serotonin syndrome/neuroleptic malignant syndrome when used concurrently with monoamine oxidase inhibitors (MAOIs) and antipsychotics.

Use in special population: In hepatic impairment use only 10 mg. No dose reduction is required in mild to moderate renal failure and no studies with respect to severe renal failure. It belongs to pregnancy category C. Caution warranted during lactation. Below 12 years of age safety is not established.

ESLICARBAZEPINE ACETATE

Introduction: This antiepileptic belongs to iminostilbene group that also comprises carbamazepine and oxcarbazepine. Prodrug is converted to active metabolite namely S-licarbazine.

Pharmacodynamics: It competitively inhibits fast voltage-gated sodium channels, stabilizing the inactivated state and the sodium-dependent release of neurotransmitters.

Pharmacokinetics: It undergoes hydrolysis to form eslicarbazepine in liver. It has a t½ similar to that of carbamazepine (8–12 hours) and it is excreted as a glucuronide. Peak plasma concentration is attained in 1–4 hours.

Uses: This drug is the FDA approved for monotherapy as well as adjunct therapy in focal epilepsies.

Dose: Ranges between 400 and 1,200 mg/day. Start with a lower dose and titrate gradually.

Adverse effects: Nausea, vomiting, dizziness, drowsiness, ataxia, and hyponatremia are common adverse effects.

Precaution: Dose reduction is necessary in patients with renal failure. It belongs to pregnancy category C and regarding lactation discontinue nursing or the drug based on the situation.

ETEPLIRSEN

Introduction: Antisense oligonucleotide (ASO) approved for Duchenne muscular dystrophy (DMD) with confirmed mutation of the *DMD* gene that is amenable to exon 51 skipping. One of the most controversial approval by the FDA in 2016. For continued approval clinical benefit must be confirmed. Eteplirsen is an ASO of the phosphorodiamidate morpholino oligomer (PMO) subclass. European medicine agency rejected this drug.

Pharmacodynamics: This ASO binds to pre messenger ribonucleic acid (mRNA) transcript and hides exon 51 from the RNA splicing machinery. This action results in restoring the reading frame thereby producing a functional protein.

Pharmacokinetics: t½ is 3-4 hours. Majority of the drug is renally excreted and not metabolized by CYP enzymes in liver.

Uses: DMD with mutation amenable to exon 51 skipping. Around 13-14% of DMD patients may benefit.

Dose: 30 mg/kg administered once weekly as a 35-60 minute IV infusion.

Adverse effects: Dizziness, vomiting, and contact dermatitis.

Use in special population: Regarding its use in pregnancy and lactation data is not available. It is not used in geriatric population as DMD is a disease of children and young adults. This drug is not studied in renal or hepatic impairment.

ETHOSUXIMIDE

Introduction: It belongs to the succinimides class and most selective for absence seizures.

Pharmacodynamics: T type currents are generated by thalamic neurons which are responsible for the 3 Hz spike and wave activity. Ethosuximide inhibits this T type current and thereby effective in absence seizures.

Pharmacokinetics: About 25% of the drug is excreted in urine and rest is metabolized by microsomal enzymes in liver. t½ is 30 hours in children. A plasma concentration of 40-100 µg/mL is sufficient for satisfactory control of absence seizures.

Uses: As a monotherapy for absence seizures.

Dose: 250 mg in children 3-6 years. Maintenance dose is 20 mg/kg. 500 mg in older children. Weekly 250 mg increment and give in divided doses to reduce nausea and vomiting.

Adverse effects: Transient leukopenia, gastrointestinal side effects include nausea, vomiting, and anorexia. Drowsiness, dizziness, lethargy, and headache are some of the CNS effects. Behavioral disturbance, restlessness, agitation, and anxiety can occur when used in children with psychiatric comorbidities.

Use in special population: Caution required when used in patients with hepatic and renal impairment. Safety not established in pediatric population <3 years.

ETIZOLAM

Introduction: It is a thienodiazepine pharmacologically related to benzodiazepine but structurally different from benzodiazepine. Thiophene ring replaces benzene ring in a benzodiazepine in this drug. It has anxiolytic, anticonvulsant, hypnotic, sedative, and skeletal muscle relaxant properties. Available in japan, Italy, and India. Not FDA approved and vulnerable to abuse as illicit preparations are dangerous.

Pharmacodynamics: It binds to GABAA receptor and increases the frequency of opening of chloride channels resulting in hyperpolarization and neuronal inhibition.

Pharmacokinetics: It has bioavailability of 93% following oral administration and reaches peak plasma concentration in 1 hour. CYP3A4 system is the major metabolic pathway. It undergoes hydroxylation and conjugation to form alpha-hydroxyetizolam which retains pharmacological effects of parent drug. Parent drug t½ is 3.4 hours whereas the metabolite mentioned earlier has t½ of 8.2 hours. CYP3A4 inhibitors increase the toxicity of the drug. CYP3A4 inducer like carbamazepine decreases the levels of etizolam.

Uses: Generalized anxiety disorder with depression, panic disorder, and insomnia.

Dose: Varies from 0.5–3 mg/day.

Adverse effects: Drowsiness, ataxia, slurred speech, asthenia, muscle weakness, withdrawal effects on sudden cessation of drugs like rebound insomnia, and confusion.

Use in special population: It is not recommended in pregnancy and lactation. It is advised not to exceed 1.5 mg/day in geriatric population. No adequate data regarding its use in liver and renal dysfunction.

EZOGABINE

Introduction: It is also known as retigabine in Europe; potassium channel opener.

Pharmacodynamics: It enhances the transmembrane currents of KCNQ family of potassium channels, thereby stabilizing resting membrane potential and reducing brain excitability.

Pharmacokinetics: Oral bioavailability is 60%. It undergoes liver metabolism and t½ is 7–11 hours. Phenytoin or carbamazepine reduces ezogabine levels.

Uses: It was initially approved for focal seizures in 18 years and older and was subsequently removed from distribution due to retinal toxicity in US. It should be used when other alternatives failed in refractory focal seizures and benefit outweighs risk.

Dose: 300 mg/day initially, then increase to 600 mg/day in a weekly increment of 150 mg/week. 1,200 mg/day is the maximum dose.

Adverse effects: Vertigo, diplopia, somnolence, cognitive impairment, and fatigue. Major adverse effects include skin discoloration, bluish pigmentation of lips, urine retention, psychosis, suicidal risk, and retinal abnormalities.

Use in special population: No adequate data regarding its use in pregnant, children, and lactating mothers.

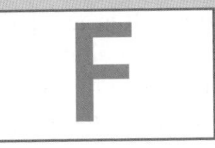

Section Outline

- Felbamate
- Fesoterodine
- Fingolimod
- Fludrocortisone
- Flumazenil
- Flunarizine
- Fluoxetine
- Flupirtine
- Folic acid
- Fondaparinux
- Fosphenytoin
- Fremanezumab
- Frovatriptan

FELBAMATE

Introduction: First second-generation antiepileptic drug (AED) approved in 1993 in US.

Pharmacodynamics: It inhibits N-methyl-D-aspartate (NMDA) evoked response, potentiates gamma-aminobutyric acid (GABA) response, and blocks sodium channel thereby contributing to wide spectrum of action.

Pharmacokinetics: It undergoes liver metabolism and half-life (t½) is 20–23 hours. It has good oral bioavailability.

Use: Focal seizures as well as generalized seizures in the setting of Lennox–Gastaut syndrome.

It is not indicated as a first-line therapy for any seizure but can be used in patients who have not responded to alternative antiseizure medications.

Dose: 600 mg 2 times a day, with subsequent titration by 600 mg to 1,200 mg/week up to 1,200 mg 3 times a day

Adverse effects: Nausea, vomiting, and anorexia are common side effects. Bone marrow suppression is of major concern. Complete blood count and liver function tests should be done prior to starting felbamate and to repeat the tests every 2 weeks in the first 6 months of treatment. Aplastic anemia (1 in 5,000–8,000) and (1 in 26,000–54,000) hepatitis are primary concerns for using this drug.

Use in special population: It is avoided in blood dyscrasias and hepatic dysfunction. It belongs to pregnancy category C and can be used only if benefits outweigh risk in pregnant patients. It is not recommended during lactation.

FESOTERODINE

Introduction: It is a prodrug that is converted to an active metabolite called 5-hydroxymethyl tolterodine (5-HMT).

Pharmacodynamics: It acts on muscarinic receptors blocking the release of acetylcholine and has some bladder selectivity.

Pharmacokinetics: It is metabolized by esterases and not by CYP2D6 unlike tolterodine. Hence, in patients with CYP2D6 polymorphism, the active metabolite HMT levels are predictable. It has a terminal t½ of 6–7 hours, hence prolonged release preparations are used.

Use: Overactive bladder.

Dose: 4 mg prolonged release once daily and maximum dose is 8 mg prolonged release once daily.

Adverse effects: Usual anticholinergic side effects include constipation, xerostomia, abdominal cramps, and blurred vision. Cognition is affected very rarely.

Use in special population: There are no controlled studies in pregnant population. Dose reduction is needed in mild-to-moderate hepatic impairment and not warranted in severe liver disease.

FINGOLIMOD

Discussed under SIP modulators.

FLUDROCORTISONE

Introduction: Synthetic steroid with maximum mineralocorticoid activity.

Pharmacodynamics: Potent mineralocorticoid and glucocorticoid activity.

Pharmacokinetics: Half-life is 3.5 hours. Biological t½ is 18–36 hours. It is metabolized in many tissues including liver.

Uses: Adrenal insufficiency, severe orthostatic hypotension.

Dose: 0.1–0.2 mg daily. Reduce to half the dose if hypertension occurs.

Adverse effects: Supine hypertension, hypokalemic alkalosis, edema and worsening of heart failure. Glucocorticoid side effects are mentioned under deflazacort.

Use in special population: No dose reduction needed in hepatic or renal failure. It belongs to pregnancy category C drug. Caution warranted in breastfeeding mom on fludrocortisone.

FLUMAZENIL

Introduction: It is imidazobenzodiazepine and a benzodiazepine antagonist.

Pharmacodynamics: It binds with high affinity to benzodiazepine binding site at GABA-A receptor and competitively blocks the allosteric effects of benzodiazepine. It also antagonizes Z drug effects. Duration of effect is 30–60 minutes.

Pharmacokinetics: It undergoes hepatic metabolism and t½ is 1 hour.

Use: Reversal of conscious sedation and anesthesia, management of benzodiazepine overdosage (the effect is incomplete and inconsistent, hence appropriate supportive measures to be taken in cases of benzodiazepine poisoning). Not effective in barbiturate, ethanol and opioid overdoses.

Dose: Only IV formulation is available. Bolus of 0.2 mg is initially given over 30 seconds and watch for improvement in consciousness. If no improvement, subsequent doses of 0.3 and 0.5 mg are used till a maximum cumulative dose of 3 mg. Additional doses may be needed in 20 minutes if sedation recurs.

Adverse effects: Headache, dizziness, and seizures.

Use in special population: It belongs to pregnancy category C. It is not recommended during labor. Caution if lactating. No dose adjustment is required in renal failure. Initial dose adjustment not needed in hepatic failure but subsequent doses may be reduced.

FLUNARIZINE

Introduction: It is a calcium channel blocker for migraine prevention (nonspecific prophylaxis). It is not approved by US FDA.

Pharmacodynamics: It blocks P/Q type calcium channel in brain and prevents cortical spreading depression. It also suppresses neurogenic inflammation by blocking release of calcitonin gene-related peptide (CGRP).

Pharmacokinetics: It has good oral bioavailability. t½ is 18 days. It undergoes hepatic metabolism. Data on elimination is not available.

Uses: Migraine prevention.

Dose: 5–10 mg/day.

Adverse effects: Weight gain, somnolence, increased appetite, and depression.

Use in special population: Not recommended in pregnancy and lactation. No adequate data in renal and hepatic impairment.

FLUOXETINE

Introduction: It is a selective serotonin reuptake inhibitor (SSRI).

Pharmacodynamics: Serotonin transporter (SERT) inhibitor. It increases concentration of serotonin in synapses as it prevents its reuptake. It does not block alpha adrenergic, histaminergic, and muscarinic receptors.

Pharmacokinetics: It has 60–80% oral bioavailability. Antidepressant effect starts from 1 to 4 weeks. It undergoes liver metabolism by CYP2D6, 2C9. t½ of parent drug is 53 hours. t½ of active metabolite norfluoxetine is 240 hours. Withdrawal syndrome is less with fluoxetine compared to other SSRI as the metabolite has long t½. It inhibits CYP2D6 and CYP3A4 to some extent.

Use: FDA approved for major depression and bulimia nervosa. It is also useful in panic disorder and premature ejaculation. Combination therapy with quetiapine is also available.

Dose: 20–80 mg is the usual dose range. Begin with 10 or 20 mg/day.

Adverse effects: Suicidal risk, worsening depression, mania, tremor, anxiety, insomnia, somnolence, flu syndrome, asthenia, nausea, vomiting, decreased libido, and delayed ejaculation.

Use in special population: Five weeks is the required time period to start MAO inhibitor in a patient on fluoxetine to avoid serotonin syndrome. For other SSRI and TCA, only 14 days gap is sufficient. It is also contraindicated in patients on concurrent thioridazine or pimozide therapy. It belongs to pregnancy category C. Half the dose is advised in liver disease. No dose adjustment is required in renal failure. In lactating mothers, it is not recommended. Safety and efficacy not established in pediatric age below 8 years.

FLUPIRTINE

Introduction: It is a triamino pyridine derivative which is an analgesic with muscle relaxant properties. It is not approved by FDA and widely used in Europe and in India.

Pharmacodynamics: It exerts glutamate antagonism through NMDAR indirectly via activating inward rectifier current K+ leading to hyperpolarization and lesser excitation of neuron. Inhibition of both mono- and polysynaptic reflexes results in muscle relaxation.

Pharmacokinetics: t½ is 6.5 hours. Oral bioavailability is 90%. It is metabolized in liver by peroxidase enzymes and 72% excreted in urine.

Uses: Acute and chronic pain conditions including fibromyalgias, tension type and migraine headaches.

Dose: It is available in oral form in strengths of 100 and 400 mg extended release preparation. Adult dose is 300–400 mg/day to a maximum of 600 mg/day. In children above 6 years, 100–150 mg/day in three divided doses.

Adverse effects: Dizziness, drowsiness, dry mouth and early satiety were the common side effects. Rash and hepatitis are serious adverse effects.

Use in special population: Half the usual dose is recommended in renal and hepatic failure patients. No adequate data to recommend in pregnancy, lactation, and children below 6 years.

FOLIC ACID

Introduction: It is a water-soluble B complex vitamin. Vitamin B9

Pharmacodynamics: Folic acid is not active as such and is converted to tetrahydrofolate which is the active form which participates in one carbon transfer reactions.

Pharmacokinetics: It has 100% bioavailability. The bioavailability of folate in food is around 50%. Metabolized and excreted in the liver and excreted in the feces.

Uses:
- Anemia, prevention of neural tube defects
- Cerebral folate deficiency
- Subacute combined degeneration

Dose:
- IV, subcutaneous, or oral
- Anemia in pediatric—0.1 mg/day in infants, 0.3 mg/day in children < 4 years, and 0.4 mg/day in children > 4 years of age.
- Anemia in adults—0.4 mg/day
- Prevention of neural tube defects—0.4-0.8 mg/day 1 month before conception and continues during first 2-3 months.
- Folinic acid for cerebral folate deficiency—0.5 mg/kg/day—2-3 mg/kg/day

Adverse effects: Avoid in known hypersensitivity and relatively nontoxic.

Use in special population: Category A in pregnancy. Distributed in to milk.

FONDAPARINUX

Introduction: Synthetic pentasaccharide that has only anti-Xa activity (1,500 Dalton molecular weight).

Pharmacodynamics: It has no intrinsic anticoagulant activity. Due to its shorter length, it cannot bind thrombin and hence has only antifactor Xa activity. Inhibiting factor Xa prevents formation of thrombin from prothrombin. Thrombin converts fibrinogen to fibrin to stabilize the clot which is halted by using fondaparinux.

Pharmacokinetics: Renal clearance is the major route. t½ is 17 hours. It is not absorbed in gastrointestinal (GI) tract hence given parenterally. Bioavailability after subcutaneous injection is 100%.

Uses: Apart from treatment of deep vein thrombosis (DVT), pulmonary embolism, acute coronary syndromes, it is also used prophylactically in critically ill patients to prevent DVT. In acute ischemic stroke, it is not regularly given but in some situations like cardioembolic strokes, cervical arteries dissection, thrombophilic conditions, stroke prevention in atrial fibrillation, and cerebral venous sinus thrombosis.

Dose: Only parenteral form is available and given subcutaneously. 5 mg (body weight <50 kg), 7.5 mg (body weight 50–100 kg), or 10 mg (body weight >100 kg) by subcutaneous injection once daily.

Adverse effects: Major bleeding, osteoporosis over long-term use (lesser risk than heparin).

Use in special population: It is drug of choice for anticoagulation during pregnancy. It is contraindicated in active bleeding, coagulopathy, recent major surgeries, acute intracranial hemorrhage, and major trauma. It is not advised in creatinine clearance <30 mL/min. Caution warranted in patients with creatinine clearance (CrCl) of 30–50 mL/min and lactating mothers. In mild-to-moderate hepatic impairment, no dose adjustment is required.

FOSPHENYTOIN

Introduction: It is hydantoin derivative; prodrug of phenytoin.

Pharmacodynamics: It binds to the active state of the sodium channel to prolong its fast inactivated state, thus reducing high-frequency firing.

Pharmacokinetics: It is highly protein bound, metabolized by CYP2C9 and CYP2C19 in liver. Its absorption is reduced by antacids and calcium. It follows nonlinear kinetics and metabolism is saturable. Toxicity occurs as drug accumulates disproportionately if exceeds therapeutic range. t½ is 12–28 hours. It is a potent enzyme inducer that reduces the efficacy of drugs metabolized by the P450 enzyme system. Fraction of free phenytoin may increase in hepatic and renal impairment.

Uses: Focal and generalized seizures. It also a second-line drug for status epilepticus.

Dose: IV formulation is used as there is less infusion site reactions and safer compared to phenytoin. 1.5 mg of fosphenytoin is equal to 1 mg of phenytoin or otherwise called as phenytoin equivalent (PE). Whenever possible, IV fosphenytoin can be replaced by oral phenytoin. IM injection is avoided in children. IV administration of fosphenytoin can be associated with hypotension and arrhythmias, so ECG and blood pressure monitoring are recommended, and the rate of IV administration should not exceed 150 mg/min for fosphenytoin. Loading dose of 15–20 mg PE/kg by IV infusion at a rate of 100–150 mg PE/minute. Maintenance dose of 4–6 mg PE/kg daily in divided doses by IV infusion is given at a rate not exceeding 150 mg PE/minute.

Adverse effects: Ataxia, drowsiness, and diplopia are common side effects. Stevens–Johnson syndrome (SJS), toxic epidermal necrolysis (TEN), acute generalized exanthematous pustulosis (AGEP), and drug reaction with eosinophilia and systemic symptoms (DRESS) are all possible severe cutaneous adverse reactions.

Use in special population: It may exacerbate generalized absence and myoclonic seizures. It is contraindicated in conduction blocks in heart. Monitor levels of phenytoin in renal failure, hepatic failure, and in pregnancy. In pregnancy, risk of congenital malformations is increased. As drug level may vary in pregnancy, patient is vulnerable to get seizures. No adequate data is available in lactating mothers.

FREMANEZUMAB

Introduction: It is recombinant humanized IgG2 monoclonal antibody specific for CGRP ligand.

Pharmacodynamics: CGRP, or calcitonin gene-related peptide, has a role in multiple pathophysiologic mechanisms underlying migraine attacks. It binds to alpha and beta isoforms of human CGRP and prevents activation of receptor. CGRP is a neuropeptide released in trigemino cervical complex system that plays a major role in cerebral vessels vasodilation and pain modulation.

Pharmacokinetics: It takes 5 days to reach maximum plasma concentration. t½ is 30 days. It undergoes probable proteolytic degradation into small peptides.

Use: Migraine prophylaxis

Dose: 225 mg subcutaneous (SC) monthly once or 675 mg SC 3 months once.

Adverse effects: Constipation and injection site reaction.

Use in special population: It has no adequate data in pregnancy. if anyone using this monoclonal antibody wants to become pregnant then a 5 months washout period is required. Pediatric safety is not established. No specific recommendations in renal, hepatic failure. Data on lactation is inadequate.

FROVATRIPTAN

Discussed under triptans.

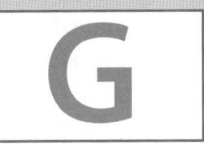

Section Outline

- Gabapentin (including gabapentin enacarbil)
- Galantamine
- Galcanezumab
- Ganciclovir
- Gepants
- Glatiramer acetate
- Givinostat
- Golodirsen
- Guanfacine

GABAPENTIN (INCLUDING GABAPENTIN ENACARBIL)

Introduction: It consists of gamma-aminobutyric acid (GABA) molecule covalently bonded to cyclohexane ring. Gabapentin enacarbil is a prodrug.

Pharmacodynamics: It binds to α2-δ1 subunit of voltage-gated calcium channel as well as potassium channels namely KCNQ2/3 and homomeric KCNQ3 and KCNQ5 channels. This causes hyperpolarization of cortical neurons leading to reduced excitability.

Pharmacokinetics: Half-life is 5–7 hours. Oral bioavailability reduces with increase in dosage because of active saturable transport system in gut. It is eliminated unchanged by kidneys. No significant interaction with other antiseizure medications except interference by antacids (antacids reduce absorption in gut).

Uses: Focal seizures, postherpetic neuralgia (FDA approved), restless legs syndrome, migraine, fibromyalgia, neuropathic pain, and alcohol withdrawal.

Dose: The recommended initial dose of gabapentin is 300–400 mg/day, to be increased by 300–400 mg every day up to 300–400 mg thrice a day. Maximum dose is 4,800 mg/day in three divided doses.

Adverse effects: Fatigue, dizziness, peripheral edema, somnolence, myoclonus, and ataxia are the adverse effects.

Precaution: It can be used in patients with hepatic impairment. Dose reduction is needed in renal failure. For creatinine clearance of 15 mL/min, 100–300 mg once daily is recommended. No adequate data is available in pregnant women and cause toxicity in animals. It secretes in breast milk and discontinue nursing or the drug. There is risk of respiratory depression in elderly. Pediatric safety below 3 years not established.

GALANTAMINE

Introduction: It is cholinesterase inhibitor.

Pharmacodynamics: Competitive inhibition.

Pharmacokinetics: It has 100% oral bioavailability. Half-life is 5.7 hours. It is metabolized by CYP2D6, CYP3A4, hence vulnerable to drug interactions.

Uses: Mild-to-moderate Alzheimer's disease

Dose: 8–12 mg twice daily for immediate release formulation and 16–24 mg/day for extended release. Start at lowest dose.

Adverse effects: Nausea, vomiting, diarrhea, and weight loss are the common side effects. It may increase acid secretion and caution warranted when used in patients with peptic ulcer disease and patients on nonsteroidal anti-inflammatory drugs (NSAIDs). Serious skin reactions have been reported.

Use in special population: It is advised not to exceed 16 mg/day in moderate hepatic impairment and moderate renal failure (9–59 mL/min). It is not recommended in severe hepatic or renal involvement (creatinine clearance <9 mL/min).

GALCANEZUMAB

Introduction: Recombinant humanized IgG4 monoclonal antibody specific for calcitonin gene-related peptide (CGRP) ligand.

Pharmacodynamics: CGRP, or calcitonin gene-related peptide, has a role in multiple pathophysiologic mechanisms underlying migraine attacks. It binds to alpha and beta isoforms of human CGRP and prevents activation of receptor. CGRP is a neuropeptide released in trigemino cervical complex system that plays a major role in cerebral vessels vasodilation and pain modulation.

Pharmacokinetics: It takes 5 days to reach maximum plasma concentration. Half-life is 27 days. It undergoes probable proteolytic degradation into small peptides.

Use: Migraine prophylaxis.

Dose: A loading dose of 240 mg subcutaneous (SC) is followed by 120 mg SC monthly once.

Adverse effects: Constipation and injection site reaction are the adverse effects.

Use in special population: There is no adequate data in pregnancy. 5 months washout period is required for pregnancy if patient is on this monoclonal antibody. Pediatric safety is not established. No specific recommendations are available in renal, hepatic failure. Data on lactation is inadequate.

GANCICLOVIR

Introduction: It is purine nucleoside analog of guanine; an antiviral drug.

Pharmacodynamics: Ganciclovir gets phosphorylated by viral and cellular thymidine kinases and form ganciclovir triphosphate which accumulates in infected cells only. This compound interferes with viral replication by inhibiting viral DNA polymerase as well as DNA chain termination thereby inhibiting viral replication.

Pharmacokinetics: Renal excretion by filtration and active tubular secretion is the major route of elimination. Half-life is 2–4 hours which is increased in renal failure.

Uses: Treatment and prophylaxis of cytomegalovirus (CMV) disease in immunocompromised patients and the management of congenital CMV disease.

Dose: In patients with normal renal function, induction is started at 5 mg/kg (given intravenously at a constant rate over 1 hour) every 12 hours for 14–21 days. For maintenance 5 mg/kg once daily for 3–6 weeks in case of CMV encephalitis.

Adverse effects: Myelosuppression, GI intolerance, headache, confusion, anxiety, hallucination, and insomnia are the adverse effects.

Use in special population: It belongs to pregnancy category C and caution warranted while breastfeeding. Dose reduction is needed in renal failure. Half the induction and maintenance dose is required in patients with creatinine clearance 50–60 mL/min. Further reduction is needed in severe renal failure. No adequate data is available in liver failure.

GEPANTS

Introduction: It is small molecule CGRP receptor antagonist. There are four gepants available in the market: Atogepant, rimegepant, ubrogepant, and zavegepant.

Pharmacodynamics: CGRP, or calcitonin gene-related peptide, has a role in multiple pathophysiologic mechanisms underlying migraine attacks. CGRP is a neuropeptide released in trigemino cervical complex system that plays a major role in cerebral vessels vasodilation and pain modulation. It binds to CGRP receptors with high affinity, blocking the binding of CGRP to the receptor and preventing subsequent receptor activation.

Use: For episodic and chronic migraine prevention (atogepant and rimegepant), acute attacks only (ubrogepant and zavegepant) **(Table 1)**.

Drug	Pharmacokinetics	Route/Dose	Remarks
Atogepant	Takes 1–2 hours to reach maximum plasma concentration. t½ is 11 hours Metabolized in liver by CYP3A4 system and majority of drug excreted in feces Strong CYP3A4 inhibitors increase levels of atogepant	Oral 60 mg oral daily, for patients prone for constipation use 30 mg. Use 10 mg daily if CYP3A4 strong inhibitors are used for episodic prevention. For chronic prevention do not use CYP3A4 strong inhibitors along with atogepant	For acute and prevention of migraine Dosage adjustment not needed in mild-to-moderate renal failure In severe renal failure, use 10 mg daily. In mild-to-moderate liver disease no dose adjustment needed. Avoid in severe liver disease. Data on pregnancy, lactation and pediatric safety inadequate
Rimegepant	CYP3A4, t½—11 hours	75 mg/dose. Not to exceed 75 mg in a day or more 18 doses in a month Available as oral dispersible tablet	Acute (approved in 2020) and prevention (2021) Dose adjustments needed in severe renal failure (CrCl <15 mL/min) and in severe liver disease

TABLE 1: Usage of gepants for migraine management.

Continued

Continued

Drug	Pharma-cokinetics	Route/Dose	Remarks
Ubrogepant	Metabolized by CYP3A4. Fecal excretion t½—5–7 hours	50 or 100 mg, 2nd dose may be repeated at least 2 hours later. Safety in treating more than 8 migraine days/month has not been established	Acute attacks only Dose modifications required in renal failure (<30 mL/min) and in severe hepatic impairment No data in pregnancy
Zavegepant	CYP3A4, t½ 6.5 hours. Biliary excretion	10 mg single dose as intranasal spray. Only use once in a day	No dose adjustment in renal failure No dose adjustments in mild/moderate liver failure No data in pregnancy and in severe liver failure

GLATIRAMER ACETATE

Introduction: Disease modifying parenteral drug approved for relapsing-remitting multiple sclerosis (RRMS) by the FDA in 1996 and expanded for its use in clinically isolated syndrome (CIS) and secondary progressive multiple sclerosis (SPMS). Glatiramer acetate (GA) is a random-sequence polypeptide consisting of four amino acids (alanine, lysine, glutamate, and tyrosine) with an average length of 40–100 amino acids. Initially, it was designed to mimic myelin basic protein (MBP).

Pharmacodynamics: It has immunomodulatory action though exact mechanism yet to be elucidated. It shifts the immune response from a proinflammatory state comprised of Th1 T-cells to regulatory, noninflammatory Th2 T-cells.

Pharmacokinetics: It undergoes hydrolysis to small peptides. There are no major drug interactions and no monitoring is required.

Uses: RRMS, CIS, and SPMS.

Dose: Subcutaneous injection at 20 mg daily or 40 mg 3 times a week.

Adverse effects: Post-injection reactions like chest pain, urticarial, and palpitations can occur which do not necessitate to stop the drug. Lipoatrophy at injection site can occur on chronic use. There is no opportunistic infection risk or malignancy risk.

Use in special population: It is safe in pregnancy and lactation. Safety and efficacy are not established in children <18 years though used off label in pediatric MS.

GIVINOSTAT

Introduction: Histone deacetylase inhibitor; FDA approved for DMD in march 2024.

Pharmacodynamics: Mechanism of action is not known. Therapeutic aim is to preserve muscle force and morphology.

Pharmacokinetics: Peak plasma concentration occurs in 2–3 hours. Bioavailability is not determined. Half-life is 6 hours. It undergoes liver metabolism and renal excretion. In vivo data not much available.

Uses: DMD aged ≥ 6 years.

Dose: Oral suspension 8.86 mg/mL.
- In children with 10–20 kg, 2.5 mL twice daily, 20–40 kg, 3.5 mL twice daily, 40–60 kg, 5 mL twice daily, 60 kg or more, 6 mL twice daily.

Adverse effects: Anemia, thrombocytopenia, neutropenia, hypertriglyceridemia, GI disturbances like nausea, vomiting, diarrhea, abdominal pain, and prolonged QT interval.

Use in special population: No safety data exists in children <6 years. No pregnancy and lactation data as DMD affects young males commonly. Hepatic impairment may increase drug exposure. No recommendation as of now in renal and hepatic failure.

GOLODIRSEN

Introduction: Antisense oligonucleotide approved for Duchenne muscular dystrophy (DMD) with confirmed mutation of the *DMD* gene that is amenable to exon 53 skipping. It is approved by FDA in 2019 based on increase in dystrophin in patients treated with this drug. For continued approval, clinical benefit must be confirmed.

Pharmacodynamics: This ASO binds to pre-mRNA transcript and hides exon 53 from the RNA splicing machinery.

This action results in restoring the reading frame thereby producing a functional protein.

Pharmacokinetics: Half-life is 3.4 hours. Majority of the drug is excreted unchanged by kidneys and not metabolized by CYP enzymes in liver.

Uses: DMD with mutation amenable to exon 53 skipping

Dose: 30 mg/kg administered once weekly as a 35–60 minute intravenous infusion.

Adverse effects: Headache, pyrexia, abdominal pain, and hypersensitivity reaction are the adverse effects.

Use in special population: Renal function to be monitored every month while administering this drug. Serum cystatin C, urine protein creatinine ratio to be measured prior to starting drug as serum creatinine is not a reliable marker in DMD. No specific dose recommendation is available for patients with renal impairment. No data regarding its use in pregnant women, lactating mothers, and patients with hepatic impairment.

GUANFACINE

Introduction: It is an alpha-2 agonist which is more selective than clonidine.

Pharmacodynamics: Similar to clonidine as it suppresses sympathetic outflow.

Pharmacokinetics: 50% is excreted unchanged in urine. Rest of the drug is metabolized by CYP3A4 microsomal system. Half-life is quite longer than clonidine (12–24 hours).

Uses: Attention-deficit hyperactivity disorder (ADHD) 6–17 years FDA approved formulation.

Dose: 1 mg daily at bed time. Maximum dose is 2 mg/day.

Adverse effects: Headache, somnolence, constipation, fatigue, and impotence (similar to clonidine) are the adverse effects.

Use in special population: CYP3A4 inhibitors or inducers usage along with guanfacine may alter the levels of the latter. It belongs pregnancy category B. Caution warranted in chronic hepatic, renal failure and lactation. Safety not established in children <12 years.

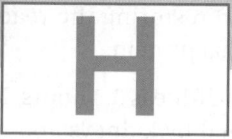

Section Outline

- Haloperidol
- Hematin
- Hydralazine
- Hypertonic saline

HALOPERIDOL

Introduction: It is butyrophenone and typical neuroleptic.

Pharmacodynamics: It blocks D2 dopamine receptors in central nervous system (CNS)

Pharmacokinetics: Oral bioavailability is 60%. Maximum concentration is reached in 2–6 hours. CYP2D6 and 3A4 enzyme metabolizes the drug. Half-life is 24 hours (12–36 hours). CYP inhibitors increase the drug levels where as inducers such as barbiturates, rifampicin, and carbamazepine reduce the drug levels by 40–70%.

Uses: Control of tics and vocal utterances of Tourette's syndrome, schizophrenia, disruptive behavior, delirium, and cancer chemo-related vomiting.

Dose: Oral tablet, intramuscular (IM), and haloperidol decanoate depot preparation are available. In children (3–12 years), usual dosage range is 0.05–0.15 mg/kg daily given in two or three divided doses. In adults, 0.5–2 mg twice or thrice oral daily. 5–20 mg is the recommended dose by the American Psychiatric Association. For severe symptoms begin at 3–5 mg twice or thrice daily. IM dose is 2–5 mg for acute agitation.

Adverse effects: Acute dystonic reaction, risk of QTc prolongation, parkinsonism, neuroleptic malignant syndrome, tardive dyskinesia, and elevated prolactin. Rarely neutropenia reported.

Use in special population: It belongs to pregnancy category C drug and breastfeeding is not recommended. No dose modification recommended in renal/hepatic failure.

HEMATIN

Introduction: It is an intravenous (IV) therapy for acute attacks of intermittent porphyria.

Pharmacodynamics: It improves symptoms by decreasing the generation of porphyrin precursors and replenishing the heme pool in hepatocytes while also downregulating delta-aminolevulinic acid synthase (ALAS1). It also induces messenger ribonucleic acid (mRNA) destabilization and blocks the mitochondrial import of the mature enzyme.

Pharmacokinetics: Metabolized in liver and enterohepatic pathway is one of the elimination route. Bilirubin metabolites are excreted in feces. No other data available regarding its pharmacokinetics.

Uses: In acute attacks of acute intermittent porphyria.

Dose: 3–4 mg/kg of heme/day for 4 days IV via large peripheral vein or central line.

Adverse effects: Fever, headache, and infusion site reaction. With recurrent IV heme therapy liver fibrosis, hepatic iron overload, thromboembolic risk (repeated IV access), and tolerance develops.

Use in special population: It belongs to pregnancy category C and not advisable in preeclampsia. There is no adequate data regarding its use in lactation.

HYDRALAZINE

Introduction: It is a 1-hydrazinophthalazine arterial vasodilator.

Pharmacodynamics: It relaxes arteriolar smooth muscle thereby reducing blood pressure (BP).

Pharmacokinetics: Oral bioavailability is 66%. Following IV, hypotensive effect starts in 5–20 minutes and lasts 2–6 hours. It is metabolized in the liver by acetylation, hydroxylation, and conjugation with glucuronic acid. Slow acetylators have high drug levels and vice versa.

Uses: BP reduction during hypertensive crisis although not favored as first-line antihypertensive.

Dose: Oral and IV formulation are available. Usual dose is 0.1–0.2 mg/kg per dose. Increase dosage up to 0.4 mg/kg per dose. It can be administered every 4 hours when given by direct IV ("bolus") injection.

Adverse effects: Common side effects include headache, tachycardia, and palpitation. It can precipitate angina and lupus.

Use in special population: Dose reduction is needed in renal failure. It belongs to pregnancy category C. Caution needed while breastfeeding.

HYPERTONIC SALINE

Introduction: It is a crystalloid solution containing sodium chloride higher than human serum. Both 3% and 5% are the Food and Drug Administration (FDA) approved.

Pharmacodynamics: It increases the osmolarity of blood. It draws fluid from extravascular space to intravascular space thereby reducing vertebral edema similar to 20% mannitol. It produces less diuresis than mannitol but increases serum sodium. It should be discontinued after symptoms resolve. It also stimulates pituitary to secrete vasopressin.

Pharmacokinetics: Not available.

Uses: The FDA has approved both 3% and 5% for reduction of intracranial pressure and hyponatremia.

Dose: It can be given as bolus or IV infusion and advised not to correct >8 mEq/L/day. This can be achieved by giving 100 mL bolus in 10 minutes interval up to 3 per day. In pediatric head injury, 6.5–10 mL/kg bolus of hypertonic saline is the recommended dose. Central vein is preferable, if not available peripheral access is accepted.

Adverse effects: Hyperchloremic metabolic acidosis, hypernatremia, IV site infusion reactions, hypervolemia, and osmotic demyelination, if sodium corrected too rapidly.

Use in special population: It belongs to pregnancy category C.

I

Section Outline

- Idebenone
- Imipramine
- Indomethacin
- Inebilizumab
- Interferon alpha
- Interferon beta
- Intravenous immunoglobulin
- Isoprinosine
- Istradefylline

IDEBENONE

Introduction: It is a synthetic analog of ubiquinone. It has antioxidant property and not FDA approved but approved by European Medicine Agency.

Pharmacodynamics: It interacts with electron transport chain, increases ATP availability for mitochondrial function, reduces free radicals, inhibits lipid peroxidation and protects mitochondria from oxidative damage.

Pharmacokinetics: It is well absorbed from gut. Within 1 hour, maximum plasma concentration is reached. It undergoes high first-pass metabolism. Metabolism is through oxidative reduction followed by conjugation to glucuronide and sulfates. Renal elimination is the major route. Details regarding half-life (t½) are not available.

Uses: Leber hereditary optic neuropathy and Friedreich ataxia.

Dose: Low dose is 5 mg/kg/day and high dose is 60 mg/kg/day in three divided doses (well tolerated in trials).

Adverse effects: Nasopharyngitis and mild diarrhea are adverse effects.

Use in special population: Details inadequate in pregnancy, lactation, hepatic and renal failure.

IMIPRAMINE

Introduction: Tricyclic antidepressant, dibenzoazepine derived.

Pharmacodynamics: Enhances norepinephrine and serotonin neurotransmission by inhibiting their reuptake into presynaptic terminal. It also blocks histamine receptor H1, alpha 1 adrenergic, muscarinic receptor too.

Pharmacokinetics: Bioavailability is 43%. Peak within 1–2 hours. Metabolized by CYP2D6, CYP1A2, and to a lesser extent by CYP3A4. Metabolites are excreted by kidneys. t½ is 8–20 hours. Antidepressant effect occurs in 1–3 weeks.

Uses: Major depression, ≥6 years nocturnal enuresis, attention-deficit hyperactivity disorder (ADHD), eating disorder, post-herpetic neuralgia, and anxiety

Dose: For depression, 50–150 mg is the maintenance dose. Start at low dose.
- For enuresis, 25 mg capsule 1 hour before bed time. Increase to 50 mg after 1 week if no response. In children >12 years, 75 mg is the maximum dose.

Adverse effects: Anticholinergic side effects include dry mouth, constipation, and tachycardia. Sedation, weight gain and orthostatic hypotension, prolonged QT interval, increased suicidal tendency, sexual dysfunction, and lower seizure threshold.
- In children when used for enuresis, it can cause nervousness, sleep disorders, and fatigue.

Use in special population: It belongs to category D, lactation not advised. In children with nocturnal enuresis below 6 years, safety not established. Contraindicated in patients who had MAOI in last 14 days and recovering phase of myocardial infarction. Use with caution in moderate-to-severe hepatic and renal failure.

INDOMETHACIN

Introduction: Indole acetic acid derivative and a reversible COX-1/COX-2 inhibitors [nonsteroidal anti-inflammatory drug (NSAID)].

Pharmacodynamics: It inhibits COX-1 and COX-2 reversibly. It has analgesic, antipyretic, and anti-inflammatory activity. The mechanism behind the therapeutic effect of indomethacin on certain headache disorders is unknown. Apart from COX inhibition, reduction of cerebral blood flow and NO inhibition.

Pharmacokinetics: Oral bioavailability is 100%. It undergoes liver metabolism and has a t½ of 7 hours and 60% of the drug undergoes renal excretion. Remaining 40% undergoes biliary excretion. It is highly lipid soluble and enter the central nervous system (CNS) easily.

Uses: Hemicrania continua and paroxysmal hemicrania, primary headache associated with sexual activity.

Dose: 25 mg orally 3 times daily for 5–7 days, followed by 50 mg 3 times daily for 5–7 days, followed by 75 mg 3 times daily for 2 weeks.
- Extended release preparation is better tolerated, but conventional preparation is efficacious.
- Rectal suppository is also available.

Adverse effects: Gastrointestinal (GI) toxicity includes irritation, bleeding, ulcer, headache, dizziness, nausea, and dyspepsia.
- Use of H2 blockers or proton pump inhibitors may be useful to circumvent GI side effect.

Use in special population: It is contraindicated in asthma, urticaria, and who have hypersensitivity to NSAIDs. Lactation is not recommended in mothers taking indomethacin. Use in second trimester can cause fetal renal dysfunction. Use in 30 or more weeks pregnant women may cause premature closure of ductus arteriosus of the fetus.

INEBILIZUMAB

Introduction: Recombinant humanized IgG1 monoclonal antibody against CD19 expressing B cells.

Pharmacodynamics: It binds to CD19 B cells and depletes them by making them undergo antibody-dependent cellular lysis.

Pharmacokinetics: Its t½ is 18 days. It undergoes proteolytic degradation into peptides.

Uses: It is designated as orphan drug by FDA for treatment of neuromyelitis optica and neuromyelitis optica spectrum disorders.

Dose: 300 mg by IV infusion, followed 2 weeks later by a second 300-mg dose by IV infusion. Subsequent dose is 300 mg every 6 months.

Adverse effects: Infusion site reactions, urinary tract infection (UTI), arthralgia, reactivation of infections like progressive multifocal leukoencephalopathy (PML), hepatitis B, and tuberculosis.

Use in special population: Tuberculosis and hepatitis B viral infection (if HbsAg negative core antibody to be tested) to be ruled out prior to starting the drug. Premedication with paracetamol, low-dose steroid, and antihistamine helps to avoid infusion-related reaction. No adequate data in pregnancy and lactation. No adequate studies in renal and hepatic impairment. Pediatric safety is not established.

INTERFERON ALPHA

Introduction: It belongs to family of glycoprotein with antineoplastic, antiviral, and immunomodulatory properties.

Pharmacodynamics: It activates natural killer (NK) cells and directly inhibits viral replication.

Pharmacokinetics: Data not available.

Uses: Hepatitis B and C, human papilloma virus, subacute sclerosing panencephalitis (SSPE) intrathecal along with isoprinosine.

Dose: Various dosing schedules are available. Gascon et al. regimen includes 1 MIU/m^2 and escalated to 10 MIU/m^2 over 5 inpatient days and then 100 MIU/m^2 twice a week for 6 months via Ommaya reservoir combined with isoprinosine.

Adverse effects: Fever, lethargy, loss of appetite, headache, myalgia, nausea, and rigors and chemical meningitis if given intrathecally.

Use in special population: It belongs to category C in pregnancy.

INTERFERON BETA

Introduction: Interferon (IFN) beta-1b was the first disease-modifying agent in multiple sclerosis in 1993. Five distinct versions are available.

Pharmacodynamics: Mechanism of action is not fully understood. It enhances the expression of the immunoregulatory cytokine interleukin-10 and soluble VCAM-1. It also reduces proinflammatory cytokines, enhances suppressor T cell activity, and reduces antigen presentation to T cells.

Pharmacokinetics: Bioavailability after subcutaneous injection is 50%. t½ for Avonex and Rebif (IFN β-1a) is 19 and 69 hours, respectively. For IFN β-1b, the t½ varies from 8 minutes to 4 hours.

Uses: It is approved for clinically isolated syndrome (CIS), relapsing-remitting multiple sclerosis (RRMS), and active secondary progressive multiple sclerosis (SPMS) in adults.

Dose: Five forms are available—
1. *Avonex*: Interferon beta-1a 30 μg injected intramuscularly once a week (initiate at 7.5 μg/week and increase by 7.5 μg every week to the target dose).
2. *Rebif*: Interferon beta-1a injected subcutaneously three times a week (22 or 44 μg per dose, begin at 4.4 or 8.8 μg for first 2 weeks and increase to half the target dose for weeks 3 and 4; from 5th week, proceed with full dose).
3. *Plegridy*: Peginterferon beta-1a injected subcutaneously every 2 weeks [Plegridy dose should be titrated, starting with 63 μg on day 1, 94 μg on day 15, and 125 μg (full dose) on day 29].
4. *Betaseron*: Interferon beta-1b injected subcutaneously every other day (0.25 mg, begin 25% of the target dose initially, increase by 25% every 2 weeks).
5. *Extavia*: Interferon beta-1b injected subcutaneously every other day (0.25 mg, begin 25% of the target dose initially, increase by 25% every 2 weeks).

Adverse effects: Depression, suicidal tendency, hepatotoxicity, leukopenia, and thrombocytopenia are the adverse effects.

Yearly complete blood count (CBC) and liver function test (LFT) monitoring is recommended. Neutralizing antibodies can form and reduce the efficacy of interferon. Flu-like illness can occur initially few hours after taking the dose that could be lessened by NSAIDs or paracetamol.

Use in special population: Safe in pregnancy and lactation. No recommendation is available regarding its use in renal and hepatic failure patients.

INTRAVENOUS IMMUNOGLOBULIN

Introduction: It is a concentrate of pooled immunoglobulins collected from healthy donors. The composition of IVIg resembles that of human plasma. IgG forms the main component with IgA and traces of other immunoglobulin classes.

Pharmacodynamics: In autoimmune conditions, antiidiotypic antibodies in IVIg bind and neutralize circulating antibodies.

Pharmacokinetics: Half-life is 3–4 weeks. There is not much data on other parameters.

Uses: Myasthenic crisis, acute attacks of primary demyelinating diseases, peripheral demyelinating diseases including GBS, CIDP, Graves' ophthalmopathy, and multifocal motor neuropathy (MMN)

Dose: 2 g/kg given over 5 days.

Adverse effects: Infusion-related side effects like fever, headache, chills, and fatigue. Serious adverse effects include aseptic meningitis, pleural effusion, hepatitis, anaphylactic reaction, rash, renal failure, thromboembolic events, and transfusion-related acute lung injury (TRALI).

Use in special population: IVIg with sugar-based stabilizers is best avoided in renal failure and diabetes patients. MMR vaccine to be avoided in children receiving IVIg for at least 9 months. Caution warranted when used in patients with preexisting renal dysfunction. It can be used in pregnancy, children, and lactating mothers. It can be given in hepatic failure but LFT to be monitored.

ISOPRINOSINE

Introduction: It was the first drug used in treatment of SSPE. Acedoben dimepranol and inosine are combined to form isoprinosine.

Pharmacodynamics: It stimulates immunity, enhances NK cell activity, and has antiviral property.

Pharmacokinetics: Plasma concentration peaks in 1 hour after oral absorption. t½ is 50 minutes. It undergoes glucuronidation and oxidation. Drug is eliminated via kidneys.

Uses: SSPE

Dose: 50–100 mg/kg/day (maximum of 3 g/day) orally in three to five divided doses as a monotherapy or combined treatment with IFN.

Adverse effects: Headache, arthralgia renal stones, nausea, raised liver enzymes, and hyperuricemia.

Use in special population: Data not available.

ISTRADEFYLLINE

Introduction: Istradefylline is an adenosine A2A receptor antagonist.

Pharmacodynamics: Adenosine A2A receptors are highly co-localized with dopamine D2 receptors in striatum. Activation of this adenosine receptor inhibits dopamine signaling. When this receptor is blocked, dopamine is boosted in striatum.

Pharmacokinetics: It undergoes oxidative metabolism by CYP1A1 and CYP3A4. Terminal t½ is 83 hours. Metabolites are excreted in feces and urine. Peak plasma concentration occurs in 4 hours.

Uses: FDA approved for Parkinson's disease as an adjunct therapy during off periods.

Dose: The FDA recommends an oral dose of 20 mg once daily with a maximum dose of 40 mg once daily.

Adverse effects: Hallucinations, nausea, vomiting, and dizziness are possible side effects.

Use in special population: In mild hepatic impairment, no need for dose adjustment. In moderate hepatic impairment, maximum dose is 20 mg. In severe hepatic impairment, it is best avoided. No adequate data in pregnancy (not recommended in pregnancy), lactation, and pediatric population.

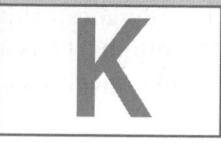

Section Outline

- Ketamine
- Ketorolac

KETAMINE

Introduction: It is an arylcyclohexylamine and congener of phencyclidine. It is available as a mixture of the R+ and S–isomers.

Pharmacodynamics: It is a N-methyl-D-aspartate (NMDA) receptor antagonist and predominantly inhibits excitatory neurotransmission at glutamatergic synapses. It increases cerebral blood flow, heart rate, mean arterial pressure, cardiac output (due to its indirect sympathomimetic effect by inhibiting catecholamine reuptake), and intracranial pressure. It produces dissociative anesthesia. It is a potent bronchodilator (useful in asthmatics) and also has analgesic activity.

Pharmacokinetics: Half-life is 2.5 hours (in children 100 minutes). It is metabolized to norketamine by hepatic CYPs (mainly by 3A4). Norketamine is hydroxylated and excreted in urine and bile.

Uses: Sedation, anesthesia, postoperative pain depression (S-enantiomer), and refractory and super-refractory status epilepticus.

Dose: Intravenous dose is 1.0–4.5 mg/kg (induction dose for anesthesia). Induction dose effect lasts 5–10 minutes. Induction dose infusion rate is 0.5 mg/kg/min.

Adverse effects: Emergence delirium (benzodiazepine concomitant administration can minimize psychotomimetic effects), hypertension, tachycardia, risk of laryngospasm, and increased intraocular pressure.

Use in special population: It is not an ideal drug for patients with ischemic heart disease as it increases myocardial oxygen consumption. No specific recommendation is available in hepatic and renal failure. It is better to avoid in liver failure. It is not recommended in pregnancy and lactation. Though safety not established in pediatric patient it is used widely in children.

KETOROLAC

Introduction: It is a reversible COX-1/COX-2 inhibitor [nonsteroidal anti-inflammatory drug (NSAID)].

Pharmacodynamics: It inhibits COX-1 and COX-2. It has analgesic, antipyretic, and anti-inflammatory activity.

Pharmacokinetics: Oral bioavailability is 80–100%. When given intramuscular (IM) it is rapidly and completely absorbed. Onset of action is in 10 minutes and analgesic effect lasts 75–150 minutes when given IM. When taken orally action starts at 30–60 minutes and peak analgesia occurs at 1.5–4 hours. It undergoes liver metabolism by hydroxylation. Half-life is 4–6 hours. Renal excretion of parent drug and metabolites constitute 92%.

Uses: Pain management including aborting acute attack of migraine.

Dose: 30 mg IV for a single dose and 60 mg IM for a single dose. Half the above dose is recommended for patients weighing <50 kg. Nasal spray available in some countries (15.75 mg per 100 µL metered spray). Oral dose is initiated at 20 mg. Subsequent doses are 10 mg not exceeding total dose of 40 per day.

Adverse effects: Gastrointestinal (GI) toxicity includes irritation, bleeding, ulcer, headache, dizziness, nausea, and dyspepsia. Use of H2 blockers or proton pump inhibitors may be useful to circumvent GI side effect.

Use in special population: It is contraindicated in asthma, urticaria, and hypersensitivity to NSAIDs. Lactation is not recommended in mothers taking ketorolac. Use in second trimester can cause fetal renal dysfunction. Use in 30 or more week's pregnant women may cause premature closure of ductus arteriosus of the fetus. Caution required when using in hepatic and renal failure patients.

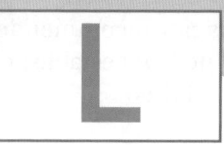

Section Outline

- Labetalol
- Lacosamide
- Lamotrigine
- Lasmiditan
- Lemborexant
- Levetiracetam
- Levodopa
- Lidocaine
- Low-molecular-weight heparin

LABETALOL

Introduction: It is a selective alpha-1 blocker and nonselective beta-blocker. The potency of the mixture for beta-adrenergic receptor blockade is 5–10 times that for alpha-1 receptor blockade. It has weak intrinsic sympathomimetic activity.

Pharmacodynamics: Alpha-1 blockade results in arterial smooth muscle relaxation and subsequent vasodilatation. Beta-1 blockade suppresses reflex sympathetic stimulation of heart. Beta-2 agonist results in vasodilation. All these actions contribute to decrease in blood pressure (BP).

Pharmacokinetics: It undergoes liver metabolism through glucuronidation. Half-life (t½) is 3–4 hours. Bioavailability is 33% due to first pass metabolism though absorbed well from gut. Intravenous (IV) formulation acts in 2–5 minutes, peaks in 5–15 minutes, and action lasts for 2–4 hours.

Uses: Hypertensive crisis in pregnancy (less placental transfer due to poor lipid solubility), most of the hypertensive emergencies except in acute heart failure. For BP reduction in acute stroke patients.

Dose: IV formulation and oral tablets are available. Initially, 100 mg twice daily, either alone or in combination with a diuretic for hypertension (oral). Direct IV at a dose of 20 mg is given for hypertensive crisis and each 10 minutes, 40–80 mg can be given till desired reduction in BP is attained (cumulative dose 300 mg). Initial rate of 2 mg/minute by continuous IV infusion can also be given as an alternate to direct IV bolus; adjust rate according to the BP response.

Adverse effects: Nausea, dizziness, and symptomatic orthostatic hypotension are common side effects. Abrupt withdrawal may exacerbate angina in coronary artery disease (CAD) patients.

Use in special population: It is contraindicated in cardiac failure, asthma, and cardiogenic shock. Once daily dose is recommended in severe renal failure. Data in hepatic impairment is not adequate, but dose reduction may be needed. It belongs to category C drug and can be used in pregnancy if benefits outweigh risk. Caution is warranted if lactating mother is taking labetalol as it can be secreted in breast milk.

LACOSAMIDE

Introduction: It is a stereoselective enantiomer of the amino acid and L-serine.

Pharmacodynamics: It enhances slow inactivation of sodium channels compared to other sodium channel blocking antiepileptics where they promote fast inactivation.

Pharmacokinetics: There is not much drug interaction when used along with other antiepileptics. Majority of the drug is excreted in urine. It has a t½ of 12–16 hours and peak plasma concentration is reached in 1–4 hours after oral ingestion. Injectable forms are also available for use.

Uses: Approved by the Food and Drug Administration (FDA) as a monotherapy and adjunctive therapy for focal-onset seizures in patients 17 years of age or older. It can be used as an off-label treatment in painful diabetic neuropathy.

Dose: As a monotherapy it is started in a dose of 50–100 mg twice a day. Increase up to 200–400 mg/day. In patients weighing <50 kg, it is started at 2 mg/kg/day in two divided doses and maintenance dose of 6–12 mg/kg/day in two divided doses.

Adverse effects: Minor adverse effects include nausea, vomiting, diplopia, sedation, and rarely suicidal ideations. No major adverse effects and has minimal hepatic metabolism. QT interval is not prolonged though PR interval is prolonged in some.

Use in special population: A quarter reduction of the dose is needed in severe renal failure. In severe hepatic disease, it is not recommended. No human studies are available for its use in pregnancy and lactation. Safety and efficacy is not established in children <4 years.

LAMOTRIGINE

Introduction: Phenyltriazine derivative initially developed as an antifolate agent.

Pharmacodynamics: Like phenytoin and carbamazepine, lamotrigine is also a sodium channel blocker, delaying the recovery from inactivation of recombinant sodium channel. It also possibly inhibits synaptic release of glutamate by acting at sodium channels themselves.

Pharmacokinetics: t½ is 24–30 hours when used as monotherapy. It undergoes glucuronidation in liver. Valproate increases the concentration of lamotrigine whereas carbamazepine and phenytoin decrease the lamotrigine level. It is excreted in urine as conjugated glucuronides. It has good oral bioavailability and only oral form is available. Therapeutic range is 2.5–15 µg/mL.

Uses: Monotherapy and add-on therapy of focal and secondarily generalized tonic-clonic seizures in adults and Lennox-Gastaut syndrome in both children and adults, neuropathy, trigeminal autonomic cephalalgia (TAC) and bipolar disorder.

Dose: Start initially at 50 mg/day for 2 weeks for patients who are on hepatic inducing drugs. The dose is increased to 50 mg twice per day for 2 weeks and then increased in increments of 100 mg/day each week up to a maintenance dose of 300–500 mg/day divided into two doses.

For patients taking *valproate* in addition to an enzyme-inducing antiseizure drug (ASD), the starting dose should be 25 mg every other day for 2 weeks, followed by an increase to 25 mg/day for 2 weeks; the dose then can be increased by 25–50 mg/day every 1–2 weeks up to a maintenance dose of 100–150 mg/day in two divided doses.

Adverse effects: Dizziness, nausea, vomiting, ataxia, blurred or double vision, and rash when lamotrigine is added to another ASD. Rash incidence is higher in children (0.8%) than in adults (0.3%).

Use in special population: Patients with mild hepatic impairment do not need dose reduction. In moderate and severe hepatic dysfunction dose reduction is necessary. In pregnancy, exposure and epidemiological studies did not show any increase in major congenital malformation. Hence, can be used in pregnancy. There can be an increase in seizure frequency during 7th month of gestation in mothers who are on lamotrigine monotherapy. It may be excreted in breast milk. Infants may be drowsy or may have poor sucking. But when the benefits of breast milk outweigh adverse effects, breastfeeding is recommended.

LASMIDITAN

Introduction: Serotonin 5-HT1F receptor agonist; lacks vasoconstrictive effects such as triptan and ergots.

Pharmacodynamics: It is a 5-HT1F agonist but exact mechanism of action not known. It probably decreases neuropeptides such as calcitonin gene-related peptide (CGRP) and substance P which have significant role in trigeminal pain pathways.

Pharmacokinetics: It is metabolized by non-CYP enzymes and renally excreted. Oral bioavailability is 40%. Pain reduction occurs in 1–2 hours. t½ is 5.7 hours.

Uses: Treatment of acute attack of migraine.

Dose: It is available as oral tablets of three strengths including 50 mg, 100 mg, and 200 mg and taken as a single dose during the headache episode. Benefit is not established if second dose taken in 24 hours.

Adverse effects: Dizziness, sedation, and bradycardia.

Use in special population: No dose reduction is needed in mild to moderate liver dysfunction or any severity of renal failure. In severe liver failure, drug is not recommended. No data regarding its usage in pregnancy and lactation. Safety is not established in pediatric population.

LEMBOREXANT

Introduction: It is orexin receptor antagonist.

Pharmacodynamics: Orexin neuropeptide plays a vital role in maintaining wakefulness. Increased orexin activity is associated with insomnia. This drug blocks orexin receptor competitively and promotes sleep.

Pharmacokinetics: t½ is 17–19 hours. It is metabolized predominantly by CYP3A4 and forms major metabolite called M10 which is also pharmacologically active. Peak concentration occurs in 1–3 hours after oral ingestion. Majority of the drug is excreted in feces.

Uses: Insomnia.

Dose: 2.5–10 mg with minimal early morning drowsiness and do not produce anterograde amnesia like the benzodiazepines or Z drugs. Start with a lower dose.

Adverse effects: Somnolence at higher doses is the common side effect. Complex sleep behaviors such as sleep walking, suicidal tendency, and sleep paralysis are also reported.

Use in special population: In elderly >65 years and in moderate hepatic impairment, 5 mg is the maximum. In severe liver disease, it is avoided. In renal failure no dose reduction is needed. It is contraindicated in narcolepsy. No data regarding its use in pregnancy and lactation. Infant to be monitored.

LEVETIRACETAM

Introduction: It is a pyrrolidine derivative.

Pharmacodynamics: It binds to SV2A affecting cellular function or neuronal excitability by modifying the release of excitatory neurotransmitter glutamate and inhibitory neurotransmitter GABA through an action on vesicular function. It also inhibits calcium fluxes from intracellular stores and via N-type calcium channels.

Pharmacokinetics: 95% of the drug is excreted in urine out of which 65% excreted unchanged. t½ is 6–7 hours. No known drug interaction as it does not induce or inhibit CYP.

Uses: FDA approved for adjunctive therapy for myoclonic, focal-onset, and primary generalized tonic–clonic seizures in adults and children as young as 4 years old.

Dose: Initiate at 500–1,000 mg/day. Every 2–4 weeks 1,000 mg is incremented to a maximum dose of 3,000 mg. It is available in solution, injectable, immediate release, and extended release oral forms.

Partial seizures in pediatric patients 1 to <6 months of age (immediate-release preparations)

Children weighing ≤20 kg should receive oral solution. Initially, 14 mg/kg daily (administered as 7 mg/kg twice daily). Increase by 14 mg/kg daily at 2-week intervals up to recommended dosage of 42 mg/kg daily (administered as 21 mg/kg twice daily).

Partial seizures in pediatric patients 6 months to <4 years of age (immediate-release preparations)

Children weighing ≤20 kg should receive oral solution; children weighing >20 kg may receive either tablets or oral solution. Initially, 20 mg/kg daily (administered as 10 mg/kg twice daily). Increase by 20 mg/kg daily at 2-week intervals up to recommended dosage of 50 mg/kg daily (administered as 25 mg/kg twice daily).

Pediatric patients weighing 20–40 kg: Initially, 500 mg daily (administered as 250 mg twice daily); may increase dosage by 500 mg daily every 2 weeks up to maximum of 1.5 g daily.

Adverse effects: Irritability and hostility occurs more often in children, somnolence, ataxia, dizziness, and asthenia.

Use in special population: No dose adjustment is needed in hepatic failure. In moderate to severe renal failure, half the dose reduction is needed and supplemental dose of 250–500 mg after dialysis is recommended. It belongs to pregnancy category C and is also secreted in breast milk. Discontinue nursing or the drug as it carries risk in newborn.

LEVODOPA

Introduction: It is a dopamine precursor and an antiparkinsonian drug. Levodopa is the levorotatory isomer of dihydroxyphenylalanine and the metabolic precursor of dopamine. Carbidopa is a decarboxylase inhibitor that inhibits the peripheral decarboxylation of levodopa to dopamine. Benserazide (50 mg) is also a decarboxylase inhibitor available with levodopa 200 mg under the trade name Madopar.

Pharmacodynamics: Striatal dopamine content is reduced to >80%, with a parallel loss of neurons from the substantia nigra, suggesting that replacement of dopamine could restore function. Levodopa increases dopamine in nigrostriatal pathway to ameliorate symptoms of Parkinson disease.

Pharmacokinetics: Peak plasma concentration is reached after oral tablet in 0.5–2 hours. It is metabolized in stomach and intestine. It passes through liver where it is decarboxylated to dopamine. It is excreted in urine as metabolites. t½ is 1.5 hours.

Uses: Parkinson's disease and other Parkinson-plus syndromes (poor therapeutic response).

Dose: Start at 25 mg carbidopa and 100 mg levodopa three times a day. Increase up to 200 mg carbidopa and 800 mg levodopa. 10 mg carbidopa with 100 mg levodopa is also available. Inhalational powder and enteral suspension form available. Controlled release form is available in 125 and 250 mg which is given at night usually in patients who have troublesome bradykinesia while waking up.

Adverse effects: Dyskinesias, hallucinations, delusion, delirium, agitation, orthostatic hypotension, sleep attack during activities of daily living (ADL), nausea, and vomiting.

Use in special population: If benefit outweighs risk it can be used in pregnancy. Caution warranted during lactation. For patients <18 years, safety is not established. Caution required in hepatic and renal failure.

LIDOCAINE

Introduction: It is an aminoethylamide used as a local anesthetic. It has a fast, long-lasting, and intense anesthesia than procaine of same concentration.

Pharmacodynamics: It blocks both open and inactivated Na$^+$ channels. Epinephrine when used along with lidocaine, reduces lidocaine toxicity and prolongs the action of lidocaine. In short-lasting, unilateral, neuralgiform headache attacks with conjunctival injection and tearing (SUNCT), sodium channel blocking action may contribute to the relief of headache.

Pharmacokinetics: It undergoes extensive first pass hepatic metabolism hence oral formulation is not useful. It undergoes dealkylation by CYP enzymes in liver to monoethylglycine and xylidide (75% excreted in urine). Terminal t½ is 1.5–2 hours.

Uses: Acute IV therapy of ventricular arrhythmias and transdermal patch for postherpetic neuralgia. For SUNCT patients are loaded with a dose of 1 mg/kg intravenously over 15 minutes. Then a continuous infusion of lidocaine in the dose of 1–4 mg/min under cardiac monitoring is given for not >7 days. Baseline electrocardiogram (ECG), renal function test (RFT), and liver function test (LFT) is a must prior to infusion. Off-label use in status epilepticus.

Dose: 2–10% solution for topical anesthesia with duration of action of ~30 minutes with a maximal healthy adult dose, ~4 mg/kg. 0.5–1% solution is used for infiltration anesthesia. For nerve blocks, epidural 1% and 2% solution are used respectively. For spinal anesthesia (lower extremity surgery) 25–50 mg is used.

Adverse effects: Common side effects include nausea, vomiting, twitching, tinnitus, drowsiness, dysgeusia, and dizziness. Serious side effects include seizure, coma, and cardiovascular depression. Paranoid ideation can be triggered and reported in SUNCT patients who were on infusion and an indication to stop the infusion.

Use in special population: Dose reduction is needed in liver failure of any severity. Dose adjustment needed only in severe renal failure. It belongs to pregnancy category B group of drugs. Caution is warranted during breastfeeding.

LOW-MOLECULAR-WEIGHT HEPARIN

Introduction: It is a biological anticoagulant that has lower molecular weight of 4,500–5,000 dalton.

Pharmacodynamics: It has no intrinsic anticoagulant activity. It binds to antithrombin and potentiates antifactor Xa activity. Inhibiting factor Xa prevents formation of thrombin from prothrombin. Thrombin converts fibrinogen to fibrin to stabilize the clot which is halted by using low-molecular-weight heparin (LMWH). It does not affect platelets or does not bind thrombin like heparin due its shorter length.

Pharmacokinetics: It undergoes renal clearance. t½ is 4 hours. It is not absorbed in gastrointestinal (GI) tract hence given parenterally. Bioavailability after subcutaneous injection is 90%.

Uses: Apart from treatment of deep vein thrombosis (DVT), pulmonary embolism, and acute coronary syndromes, it is also used prophylactically in critically ill patients to prevent DVT. In acute ischemic stroke, it is not regularly given but in some situations such as cardioembolic strokes, cervical arteries dissection, thrombophilic conditions, stroke prevention in atrial fibrillation. During the acute phase of cerebral venous thrombosis it is given subcutaneous.

Dose: Only parenteral form is available. Enoxaparin is given at a dose of 1.5 mg/kg/day or 1 mg/kg/BID subcutaneous for therapeutic purpose. Prophylactic enoxaparin is 40 mg/day. Therapeutic monitoring of anti-Xa activity is recommended in obese people [body mass index (BMI) > 40], pregnant women, children, and in renal failure patients.

Adverse effects: Major bleeding is the common side effect. Protamine sulfate is the antidote which can partially act on LMWH. Osteoporosis can occur over long-term use but has less risk than heparin.

Use in special population: It is the drug of choice for anticoagulation during pregnancy. It is contraindicated in active bleeding, coagulopathy, recent major surgeries, acute intracranial hemorrhage, and major trauma. In patients with creatinine clearance of <30 mL/min, use 1 mg/kg of enoxaparin once daily (therapeutic purpose). For prophylaxis do not exceed 30 mg/day.

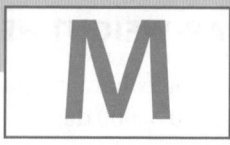

Section Outline

- Magnesium sulfate
- Mannitol
- Meclizine
- Melatonin
- Memantine
- Methotrexate
- Methylphenidate
- Methylprednisolone
- Mexiletine
- Midazolam
- Midodrine
- Milnacipran
- Mirabegron
- Mirtazapine
- Mitoxantrone
- Modafinil
- Morphine
- Mycophenolate mofetil

MAGNESIUM SULFATE

Introduction: Electrolyte, cofactor for various biochemical reactions, anticonvulsant when given parenterally.

Pharmacodynamics: Its vascular effects include smooth muscle relaxation, vasodilation by antagonizing calcium channel activity, decreased platelet aggregation, increased nitric oxide. It also decreases blood-brain barrier disruption, limits cerebral edema and decreased aquaporin 4 (AQP4) expression.

It also exhibits antiseizure mechanism, increases seizure threshold by antagonizing N-methyl-D-aspartate receptor (NMDAR) leading to limited glutamatergic (excitatory) effect.

Pharmacokinetics: By IV administration, onset of action is immediate and duration of action lasts 30 minutes. It is excreted by kidneys.

Uses: Seizure prevention and control in preeclampsia or eclampsia. It can be used parenterally for seizures due to other etiologies. Other uses include tocolytic therapy in preterm labor, repletion in total parenteral nutrition, ventricular arrhythmias, barium poisoning, and acute asthma.

Dose: In eclampsia, IV loading dose of 4–6 g, followed by a maintenance IV infusion of 1–2 g/hour for ≥24 hours. Maximum dose is 30–40 g daily.

For severe deficiency: 5 g (~40 mEq) added to 1 L of 5% dextrose injection or 0.9% sodium chloride injection infused slowly over 3 hours. Do not exceed 150 mg/min. Maximum IV concentration is 200 mg/mL. Check for knee jerk before each dose. If absent do not give additional magnesium. Respiratory rate should be above 16/min and make sure whether urine output is 100 mL or more 4 hours preceding each dose.

Adverse effects: Hypermagnesemia and respiratory depression (calcium gluconate is the antidote). Toxic effects of magnesium start at serum level of >4 mEq/L. Neurological effects include flaccid weakness, lethargy, confusion, and depression of deep tendon reflexes. Hypotension, hypoventilation, and circulatory collapse are some cardiorespiratory adverse effects.

Use in special population: In renal impairment, do not exceed 20 g/day. It is contraindicated as a parenteral administration in heart block or myocardial damage. It should not be given intravenous, 2 hours preceding delivery.

MANNITOL

Introduction: Hexacarbon, linear simple sugar.

Pharmacodynamics: Mannitol increases the serum osmolality and draws water out of brain as it cannot cross blood–brain barrier. Then it gets excreted along with the water by kidneys. Mild diuresis ensues. Similar mechanism operates in increased intraocular pressure.

Pharmacokinetics: Orally, the absorption is poor. Hence, given only IV as it gets rapidly excreted in kidneys. Intracranial pressure (ICP) starts to reduce in 15–30 minutes after IV. Effect lasts for 1.5–6 hours. It is predominantly metabolized to fructose-6-phosphate and minimal glycogen. Half-life ($t_{1/2}$) is 0.5–2.5 hours in normal renal function individuals, whereas it is 6–48 hours in renal failure patients.

Uses: FDA approved for reducing intracranial pressure associated with cerebral edema and intraocular pressure. Inhalation of the powder form of mannitol in cystic fibrosis as an adjunctive therapy is also FDA approved.

Dose: 0.25–2 g/kg, administered intravenously over 30–60 minutes.

Adverse effects: Dehydration, heart failure, hyponatremia, hypokalemia, and hypocalcemia are the adverse effects.

Use in special population: No dose reduction is required in hepatic impairment. Prior correction of electrolyte imbalance before mannitol is a must in renal impairment. It can be used in pregnancy only if benefit outweighs the risk as mannitol crosses placental barrier. No adequate data regarding its use in lactation. Children < 2 years are at increases risk of fluid electrolyte imbalances. Concurrent administration of nephrotoxic drugs is not recommended. It is contraindicated in anuria, pulmonary edema, severe dehydration, heart failure, and active intracranial bleeding.

MECLIZINE

Introduction: It is a piperazine derivative used for symptomatic treatment of vertigo.

Pharmacodynamics: Anticholinergic, antiemetic, antispasmodic, and antihistaminic activity of this drug suppresses the labyrinth excitability and conduction in vestibular–cerebellar pathways.

Pharmacokinetics: Duration of action is 12–24 hours. Metabolism of the drug is not known. Half-life is 6 hours.

Uses: Symptomatic management of vertigo in vestibular disorders and in prevention of motion sickness.

Dose: Oral formulation in a dose of 25–50 mg 1 hour before journey is recommended to prevent motion sickness. Maximum dose is 100 mg.

Adverse effects: These are drowsiness, dry mouth, and fatigue.

Use in special population: It belongs to pregnancy category B and secreted in breast milk. Discontinue nursing or the drug based on the situation. No safety data for use in children below 13 years. Alcohol intake aggravates central nervous system (CNS) depression. Avoid operating machinery and driving during drug intake.

MELATONIN

Introduction: It is a circadian signaling molecule formed in pineal gland by N acetylation and O methylation of serotonin.

Pharmacodynamics: Melatonin interacts with supra-chiasmatic nuclei of hypothalamus and retina. It acts via

MT1 and MT2 receptors and regulates sleep–wake cycle by inhibiting wake signals as well as promoting sleep signals.

Pharmacokinetics: Metabolized by CYP system hence drug interactions are quite common. Half-life ranges from 47 to 61 minutes. Oral bioavailability is 15%.

Uses: Insomnia, circadian rhythm disorders, jet lag, and shift work disorder.

Dose: Low dose 1–3 mg/day 30 minutes before bed time in children and adolescents for insomnia. For adults, 3–5 mg in the evening is recommended for insomnia for 4 weeks. For jet lag, 0.5–3 mg preflight and 5 mg postflight for 4 days. Oral tablets, oral liquids, rectal suppositories, and transdermal patches are all available.

Adverse effects: Nausea, vomiting, drowsiness, nightmares, excess daytime somnolence, and headache are the adverse effects.

Use in special population: More research required regarding its use in pregnancy and lactation. Caution warranted in hepatic and renal impairment. It is contraindicated in autoimmune diseases.

MEMANTINE

Introduction: It is a noncompetitive antagonist of N-methyl-D-aspartate receptor (NMDAR).

Pharmacodynamics: It blocks pathologic activation of NMDAR by glutamate but permits physiological activation involved in learning and memory.

Pharmacokinetics: Peak plasma concentration is attained in 3–7 hours after oral ingestion. Half-life is 60–80 hours. It is predominantly eliminated by kidneys.

Uses: Moderate-to-severe dementia (delays progression temporarily).

Dose: Initially 5 mg/day. Then increase the dose by 5 mg every week to a target dose of 10 mg twice daily. It is also available in fixed dose combination with donepezil.

Adverse effects: Constipation, dizziness, headache, and confusion.

Use in special population: 50% dose reduction (5 mg twice daily) needed in renal failure. No dose adjustment required in hepatic impairment. No data in regarding its usage in children, pregnant, and lactating mothers.

METHOTREXATE

Introduction: It is a folic acid analog and an antimitotic agent.

Pharmacodynamics: It inhibits dihydrofolate reductase (DHFR) enzyme that converts dihydrofolate to tetrahydrofolate which is essential for DNA and RNA synthesis as it acts as cofactor for purine ribonucleotides synthesis.

Pharmacokinetics: There is an initial rapid distribution, followed by renal clearance (t½ 2–3 hours). Terminal t½ is 8–10 hours and responsible for bone marrow toxicity, skin, and gastrointestinal side effects. Third spacing of fluids acts as reservoir for methotrexate and can result in toxicity. Sulfonamides, salicylates, tetracycline, chloramphenicol, and phenytoin can all displace methotrexate from albumin and can result in toxicity when used concomitantly.

Uses: Used as immunosuppressant (steroid sparing) in autoimmune diseases like rheumatoid arthritis, psoriasis, inflammatory bowel disease, etc., and an antimetabolite in chemotherapy for various malignancies. Granulomatosis with polyangiitis, inflammatory myositis, vasculitis, and myasthenia gravis are some neurological indications.

Dose: Given as oral pulse weekly. 5 mg/week initially and increase every week 2.5 mg to the desired clinical effect. Folate supplementation with 1 mg/day or 5 mg once weekly should be considered for all patients to prevent bone marrow toxicity. Weekly complete blood count (CBC), liver function test (LFT), and renal function test (RFT) to be done in the 1st month of therapy and then bimonthly at least.

Adverse effects: Common gastrointestinal (GI) side effects include nausea, vomiting, diarrhea, and mucosal ulcers.

Side effects of concern include alopecia, rash, fever, reactivation of tuberculosis, hepatotoxicity, leukopenia, GI bleed, bone marrow suppression (aplastic anemia), and renal failure.

Use in special population: Contraindicated in pregnancy and lactation as it belongs to category X. Also contraindicated in renal and hepatic impairment.

METHYLPHENIDATE

Introduction: It is a piperidine derivative which is also structurally related to amphetamine. It is a mild CNS stimulant and has more effects on mental than motor activities. Dexmethylphenidate is the d-threo-enantiomer of racemic methylphenidate. It is FDA approved for the treatment of attention-deficit hyperactivity disorder (ADHD). Both drugs have abuse potential.

Pharmacodynamics: Similar to amphetamine.

Pharmacokinetics: Half-life is 4–6 hours, orally absorbed well and reaches peak plasma concentration in 2 hours. It is metabolized by deesterification and excreted in urine as ritalinic acid.

Uses: Treatment of narcolepsy and ADHD.

Dose: Conventional and extended release oral preparations are available. Start at 5 mg twice daily and increment 5 mg every week to a maximum of 60 mg. Conventional tablets are given twice or thrice daily. Extended release is given once daily and is available in 18 mg, 36 mg, and 54 mg. Do not exceed 72 mg in extended release preparations.

Adverse effects: Common side effects include anorexia, vomiting, and weight loss. CNS adverse effects include insomnia, restlessness, headache, irritability, and anxiety. Tachycardia, palpitations, and hypertension are some cardiovascular effects.

Use in special population: Contraindicated in glaucoma and recent ingestion of MAO-B inhibitors (within 14 days of intake; risk of hypertensive crisis). It is not recommended in pregnancy. Lactation can be continued but infant to be monitored for side effects. Safety not established in children <6 years.

METHYLPREDNISOLONE

Introduction: Synthetic glucocorticoid with good anti-inflammatory potency with minimal sodium retaining capacity.

Pharmacodynamics: It has immunosuppressant action by reducing the action of lymphocytes. It reduces inflammation by inhibiting macrophages, reducing WBC adhesion to capillary endothelium, reduces capillary wall permeability and stabilizing WBC lysosomal membranes. It also antagonizes histamine.

Pharmacokinetics: Duration of anti-inflammatory action is 12–36 hours. Half-life is 2.5–3.5 hours. Metabolized predominantly in liver by CYP3A4 system.

Uses: Acute treatment for various neurological diseases including optic neuritis, CIDP, NMO, MS, inflammatory myositis, giant cell arteritis, ADEM, acute spinal cord injury, and myasthenia gravis.

Dose:
- Available in oral and injectable forms. Intravenous form in the dose of 1–1.5 g/day for 3–5 days infusion is considered as pulse therapy.
- Methylprednisolone sodium succinate (30 mg/kg initially followed by an infusion of 5.4 mg/kg/h for 23 hours) is given in acute spinal cord injury.

Adverse effects: Mood and behavior disturbance, adrenocortical insufficiency on withdrawal, hypokalemia, salt and water retention, hyperglycemia, Cushing syndrome, infections like HSV and VZV, decreased bone mineral density, avascular necrosis, myopathy, serious skin rashes, cataract, and bruising.

Use in special population: Intramuscular injection to be avoided in ITP. Metabolic clearance may be reduced in hypothyroidism and increased in hyperthyroidism. In pregnancy use if benefits outweigh risk. Discontinue nursing or the drug during lactation period. Caution warranted in osteoporosis and renal failure. Liver cirrhosis patients may show exaggerated response.

MEXILETINE

Introduction: It is an analog of lidocaine designed to reduce first-pass metabolism and belongs to class IB antiarrhythmic drugs.

Pharmacodynamics: It is a sodium channel blocker that enhances fast inactivation of sodium channels. This abolishes abnormally persistent sodium currents leading to repetitive firing of muscle fibers and myotonia.

Pharmacokinetics: It has 90% oral bioavailability and a t½ of 10–12 hours. It reaches peak concentration in 2–3 hours. It undergoes CYP metabolism hence inducers reduce drug levels whereas inhibitors increase. It has less first-pass metabolism compared to lignocaine.

Uses: Symptomatic relief for myotonia and diabetic neuropathy (off label) apart from its use in ventricular arrhythmias.

Dose: Oral 150–200 mg three times a day for myotonia and not to exceed 1.2 g in diabetic neuropathy (off-label).

Adverse effects: Tremor and nausea are the most common adverse effects. It has to be taken along with food. It has arrhythmogenic potential. Hepatotoxicity, hematotoxicity (leukopenia, thrombocytopenia), and exacerbation of heart failure are some worrisome adverse effects.

Use in special population: Dose reduction needed in hepatic impairment. It can be used in renal failure without dose reduction. It is contraindicated in AV blocks. It belongs to category C in pregnancy. Advised in lactation mothers only if breastfeeding benefits outweigh the risk.

MIDAZOLAM

Introduction: It is a short-acting benzodiazepine.

Pharmacodynamics: It binds to GABA-A receptor and increases the frequency of opening of chloride channels resulting in hyperpolarization and neuronal inhibition.

Pharmacokinetics: It has poor oral absorption and a half-life of 1.5–2.5 hours. It is metabolized through CYP450 enzymes and glucuronide conjugation. Hence vulnerable to drug interactions. Half-life is prolonged in geriatric patients.

Uses: Available in oral, buccal, nasal, and IV forms. It is used in status epilepticus (bolus as first-line drug, continuous infusion as a third-line drug), preoperative sedation and anesthesia, sedation in critical care settings

Dose:
- 0.05–0.1 mg/kg as a IV bolus dose for children between 6 months and 5 years of age (maximum 6 mg).
- 0.025–0.05 mg/kg IV for 6–12 years (maximum dose 10 mg)
- For adults, IV dose is 0.05–0.15 mg/kg and intramuscular dose in 0.07–0.08 mg/kg

Adverse effects: Nausea, vomiting, hiccough, falls, drowsiness, ataxia, and anterograde amnesia. Rapid IV administration causes hypotension, tachycardia, and respiratory depression.

Use in special population: It is contraindicated in hypotension, acute angle closure glaucoma, and shock. Even at therapeutic dosages, concurrent use of midazolam and other CNS depressants can cause fatalities and severe respiratory depression. It is avoided in pregnancy and belongs to category D. Caution warranted in breastfeeding mothers taking midazolam. Dose reduction needed in geriatric, liver disease, and renal failure.

MIDODRINE

Introduction: Sympathomimetic agent which is an alpha-1 selective agonist.

Pharmacodynamics: Desglymidodrine, an active metabolite of midodrine, acts on peripheral α-adrenergic receptors of the arterial and venous vasculature, increases the peripheral resistance and vascular tone. End result is increase in systolic blood pressure (SBP) and diastolic blood pressure (DBP).

Pharmacokinetics: It undergoes deglycination to form active metabolite desglymidodrine. It has a good oral bioavailability of 93%. 10–30 mm Hg of increase in BP noted after 1 hour of intake. Half-life is 2–3 hours.

Uses: Orthostatic hypotension.

Dose: Initially 2.5 mg three times a day and maximum of 10 mg three times a day.

Adverse effects: Supine hypertension and urinary retention.

Use in special population: 2.5 mg thrice daily recommended in renal failure. No specific recommendation in hepatic impairment. It belongs to category C drug. It is contraindicated in severe heart disease, thyrotoxicosis, and pheochromocytoma.

MILNACIPRAN

Introduction: It is a selective serotonin and norepinephrine reuptake inhibitor (SNRI).

Pharmacodynamics: SNRI that inhibits the reuptake of both norepinephrine and serotonin. It has higher selectivity for norepinephrine transporter than duloxetine or venlafaxine.

Pharmacokinetics: Oral bioavailability is 85–90%. Maximum plasma concentration is reached in 2–4 hours following intake. Glucuronide conjugation and renal excretion (90%) are the major metabolic pathways. Terminal half-life is 6–8 hours.

Uses: Fibromyalgia, off-label use in depression.

Dose: Oral form is available. Initiate at a dose of 12.5 mg/day, then increase to 12.5 mg twice daily on day 2 and day 3. Increase to 25 mg twice daily on day 4–7. After a week, maintenance dose is 50 mg twice daily. Based on clinical response, titrate. Maximum dose is 200 mg/day.

Adverse effects: Insomnia, elevated liver enzymes, headache, constipation, hyperhidrosis, nausea, vomiting, tachycardia, hypertension, withdrawal effects like irritability, anxiety and confusion. Serotonin syndrome risk is present if taken with MAO inhibitors. Suicidal tendency and worsening of depression may be seen in young adults and adolescents.

Use in special population: It is contraindicated in angle closure glaucoma, children <18 years (lack of establishment of safety), end-stage renal disease, chronic alcoholism, and chronic hepatitis. In CrCl 5–29 mL/min, use 50% of the usual dose. No dose reduction is needed in mild-to-moderate hepatic disease. It belongs to category C drug. Caution warranted while breastfeeding.

MIRABEGRON

Introduction: It is β3-selective adrenergic receptor agonist.

Pharmacodynamics: Beta-3 receptor activation in bladder wall leads to detrusor relaxation and increased bladder capacity.

Pharmacokinetics: As a result of its CYP2D6 inhibiting nature, increased levels of digoxin, metoprolol, and desipramine occur when given concomitantly. Peak plasma concentration is reached in 3.5 hours. Bioavailability is 29% for 25 mg and 35% for 50 mg. Half-life is 50 hours. It undergoes hepatic metabolism via numerous pathways involving oxidation, dealkylation, glucuronidation, and hydrolysis.

Uses: Overactive bladder symptoms like urgency, frequency, and urge incontinence. Symptomatic improvement starts after 4 weeks.

Dose: Start with 25 mg once daily and increase up to 50 mg daily.

Adverse effects: Urinary tract infection, headache, and hypertension

Use in special population: In mild hepatic impairment, mild and moderate renal failure no need dose adjustment. In moderate hepatic impairment, 25 mg is the maximum dose. In severe hepatic and end-stage renal disease (ESRD) creatinine clearance (CrCl <15 mL/min), it is best avoided. In severe renal impairment CrCl 15–29 mL/min, 25 mg can be used. Pediatric safety is not established. It belongs to pregnancy category C group of drugs. Discontinue nursing or drug during lactation period.

MIRTAZAPINE

Introduction: It is noradrenergic and specific serotonergic antidepressant (NaSSA); tetracyclic antidepressant; a piperazinoazepine derivative.

Pharmacodynamics: It blocks presynaptic alpha-2 adrenergic receptors increasing release of serotonin and norepinephrine. It also blocks histamine H1 receptor, 5-HT2A and 5-HT3 serotonin receptor subtypes.

Pharmacokinetics: Oral bioavailability is 40–60%. It reaches peak plasma concentration in 1.5 hours. Elimination half-life is 16–30 hours. It undergoes liver metabolism by CYPs2D6, 1A2, and 3A4.

Uses: Major depressive disorder.

Dose: Begin with 15 mg/day. Increase weekly or biweekly till the desired response occurs up to a maximum dose of 45 mg.

Adverse effects: Weight gain, increased appetite and sedation.

Agranulocytosis is a rare occurrence.

Use in special population: Though there is decreased clearance in renal and hepatic impairment, no specific dose recommendation is available at this time. In geriatric population too, clearance is decreased. Caution is warranted in nursing mothers and elderly people >65 years.

MITOXANTRONE

Introduction: It is synthetic anthracenedione and an anticancer drug which is a DNA replication inhibitor.

Pharmacodynamics: It interferes with topoisomerase II function thereby preventing relegation of breaks in DNA strand. It also inhibits T cell, B cell, and macrophages.

Pharmacokinetics: It has a median half-life of around 75 hours. Metabolism is not clear. A quarter of the drug is excreted in feces by hepatobiliary system and 10% in urine.

Uses: Secondary progressive multiple sclerosis (SPMS), acute myeloid leukemia, and prostate cancer.

American Academy of Neurology recommends the usage of this drug only if benefit outweighs risk in MS due to its toxicity profile.

Dose: 12 mg/m^2 once every 3 months, intravenous infusion over 15 minutes. Maximum cumulative lifetime dose is 140 mg/m^2.

Adverse effects: Nausea, vomiting, alopecia, ovarian failure, male infertility, mucositis, and myelosuppression.

Long-term use results in cardiotoxicity and chronic myeloid leukemia.

Use in special population: It is not recommended during pregnancy as it belongs to category D. Discontinue drug or nursing during lactation. In multiple sclerosis (MS) patients with hepatic impairment, drug is not recommended. No data regarding its use in renal impairment is available.

MODAFINIL

Introduction: It is a CNS stimulant to promote wakefulness. Modafinil is racemic mixture of R and S enantiomer in 50:50 ratio. Armodafinil is R enantiomer of modafinil.

Pharmacodynamics: Exact mechanism of action of modafinil for narcolepsy is not known. It weakly inhibits dopamine reuptake. It also activates excitatory glutamate circuits and inhibits GABA.

Pharmacokinetics: It is partially metabolized by CYP3A4 enzymes and rest by oxidation, hydroxylation, and glucuronide conjugation. Renal elimination constitutes 80%. Peak concentration after oral ingestion is attained in 2–4 hours. Half-life is 10–15 hours.

Uses: Narcolepsy, ADHD, off-label use in cocaine and amphetamine withdrawal. Armodafinil improve wakefulness in shift workers and in patients with obstructive sleep apnea syndrome.

Dose: 200 mg/day modafinil (maximum 400 mg/day). Armodafinil is started at a dose of 75 mg/day. Gradually increase to 150 mg/day (maximum 250 mg/day).

Adverse effects: Anxiety, insomnia, headache, nausea, rarely transient psychosis including delusions, hallucination, and mania.

Use in special population: Dose reduction is needed in patient with severe hepatic impairment (100 mg/day). It belongs to pregnancy category C. Caution warranted while breastfeeding. Safety not established below 17 years of age.

MORPHINE

Introduction: It is phenanthrene derivative which is an opioid agonist.

Pharmacodynamics: Agonist activity at mu or kappa receptor results in analgesia, sedation, respiratory depression, and constipation.

Pharmacokinetics: Oral bioavailability is around 20–40%. Metabolized in liver and conjugation with glucuronic acid. It is excreted in urine mainly as metabolites. Terminal half-life is 1.5–2 hours for intravenous form.

Uses: Cancer pain, relief of pain, and anxiety related to acute coronary syndrome

Dose:
- Oral, rectal, IV, IM, intrathecal, or epidural routes are available. Morphine sulfate in dose of 2, 4, 5, 8, and 10 mg/mL injections are available in single-dose prefilled syringes for direct IV or IM injection.
- For pediatric patient, 15 mg oral every 4 hours as needed for pain and try to use lowest effective dosage.
- For adults, 15–30 mg oral every 4 hours as required.
- 0.1–0.2 mg/kg every 4 hours as needed by slow IV injection
- In patients with acute myocardial infarction (STEMI), initial IV dose of 2–4 mg is recommended; additional doses of 2–8 mg may be administered every 5–15 minutes as required.

Adverse effects: Respiratory depression, risk of addiction, abuse, misuse, withdrawal effects on abrupt discontinuation, cardiovascular instability, and increased risk of seizures. Rapid IV may result in chest wall rigidity.

Common side effects include constipation, sedation, dizziness, vomiting, headache, and diaphoresis.

Use in special population: Lower than usual dosage is advised in liver failure and renal failure patients, geriatric patients (as they have increased sensitivity). It is contraindicated in asthma, respiratory depression, and MAOI intake within last 14 days. Concomitant use with benzodiazepine results in profound sedation and coma. It is not recommended in pregnancy and lactation. It can prolong labor.

MYCOPHENOLATE MOFETIL

Introduction: It is 2-morpholinoethyl ester of mycophenolic acid (MPA).

Pharmacodynamics: Prodrug is converted to MPA. It inhibits inosine monophosphate (IMP) dehydrogenase reversibly in a selective and noncompetitive manner. IMP dehydrogenase is essential for de novo synthesis of guanine nucleotide. By inhibiting this pathway, T and B lymphocyte proliferation and functions are affected including antibody formation, adhesion, and cellular migration.

Pharmacokinetics: It undergoes glucuronidation and converted to MPA glucuronide. MPA and MPA glucuronide levels are increased in patients with renal impairment. Half-life is about 16 hours. Antacids and cholestyramine decrease drug absorption. When used with acyclovir, both the drug levels increase.

Uses: It is used as a steroid-sparing agent in myasthenia gravis, immune mediated neuropathies, and inflammatory myositis.

Organ transplant recipients receive mycophenolate mofetil (MMF) to prevent rejection in combination with other immunosuppressants.

Dose:
- Initiate at a dose of 250–500 mg/day. Increase 500 mg every week to reach a target dose of 2–3 g. Oral tablet, solution, and intravenous formulation are available.
- 600 mg/m^2 as the oral suspension twice daily (maximum 1 g twice daily) is the recommended dose for oral formulation in pediatric population.

Adverse effects: Hematological side effects include pure red cell aplasia and neutropenia. Nausea, vomiting, and diarrhea are some of the GI adverse effects. Risk of progressive multifocal leukoencephalopathy (PML), cytomegalovirus infection, lymphomas, and skin malignancies are increased when used with other immunosuppressant.

Use in special population: It is contraindicated in pregnancy as it is a category D drug having teratogenic potential. It can be used in pediatric population as early as 3 months of age. Avoid breastfeeding for at least 6 weeks after discontinuing mycophenolate sodium. Oral solution contains aspartame hence caution is warranted when using in children with phenylketonuria. No dose recommendation is available for hepatic and renal impairment. However, it is advised not to exceed 2 g/day in severe renal impairment.

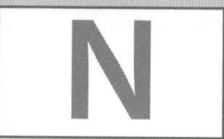

Section Outline

- Naloxone
- Naltrexone
- Naproxen
- Natalizumab
- Neostigmine
- Nicergoline
- Nimodipine
- Nortriptyline
- Nusinersen

NALOXONE

Introduction: Naloxone is an opioid receptor antagonist used to rapidly reverse opioid action in cases of opioid poisoning.

Pharmacodynamics: It is an inverse agonist at opioid receptor more specifically at the μ receptor. Hence, it is used for rapid reversal of opioid toxicity as it is very short acting. It can precipitate opioid withdrawal in tolerant patients.

Pharmacokinetics: Available as intramuscular, intravenous, subcutaneous, or intranasal forms. Has wide volume of distribution. Metabolized by glucuronidation in the liver and is excreted in the urine. Half-life (t½) is 1.8–2.7 hours.

Uses:
- Rapid reversal of opioid poisoning when used as intravenous or intranasal route
- Used sublingually with buprenorphine in treatment of opioid dependence
- Off-label use in opioid-induced pruritus

Dose:
- Toxicity in opioid-dependent patients—0.04–0.1 mg
- Toxicity in opioid-nondependent patients—0.4 mg
- Large initial dose—1–2 mg may be given in apneic patients
- Intranasally—4 mg in a single spray (mostly in out of hospital settings), repeat doses, every 2–3 minutes may be given in alternate nostrils

Adverse effects:
- Precipitation of opioid withdrawal
- Noncardiogenic pulmonary edema (persistent hypoxic despite resolution of respiratory depression with pink frothy sputum)

Use in special population: It is the recommended agent for opioid toxicity in pregnancy. Produces improvement in chronic kidney disease-induced pruritus.

Nalorphine

Nalorphine is a mixed opioid agonist and antagonist. It acts as antagonist at μ receptor and agonist at κ receptor.

NALTREXONE

Introduction: It is a relatively pure synthetic congener of oxymorphone and long-lasting opioid antagonist. Its primary use is in morphine de-addiction but also used for alcohol de-addiction.

Pharmacodynamics: It is an opioid receptor antagonist at μ, κ, and δ receptors in the central nervous system (CNS), with the highest affinity for the μ receptor. Hence, it blocks most effects of opioids.

Pharmacokinetics: Once ingested, it is absorbed in the gastrointestinal (GI) tract and metabolized in the liver to 6-β-Naltrexol. The long-acting properties of naltrexone are due to this metabolite. Naltrexone has a t½ of 4 hours but to 6-β-Naltrexol has a t½ of 13 hours.

Uses:
- Opioid de-addiction
- Alcohol de-addiction since the effects are mediated through opioid receptor. Important point to remember is to start naltrexone only after a period of abstinence of at least 3 days since it can precipitate acute withdrawal symptoms when started early.

Dose: 50 mg/day. Start at 12.5 or 25 mg in patients with higher risk of adverse effects (woman, younger patients, and patients with shorter abstinence).

Adverse effects:
- Common—nausea, vomiting, headache, dizziness, and somnolence
- Less common—diarrhea, rash, stomach pain, chest pain, constipation, mild depression, and delayed ejaculation

Use in special population: Needs careful monitoring and dose reduction in liver and renal failure. Not to be used in pregnancy (category C). To be avoided in woman of childbearing age.

NAPROXEN

Introduction: Naproxen is a nonsteroidal anti-inflammatory drug (NSAID), which is the Food and Drug Administration (FDA) approved for acute gout, ankylosing spondylitis, osteoarthritis (OA), tendonitis, etc. Its use in migraine is off-label but is considered the first-line abortive medication in migraine.

Pharmacodynamics: Naproxen is a NSAID, hence inhibits cyclooxygenase-1 and 2 (COX-1 and 2). These are enzymes which catalyze breakdown of arachidonic acid to prostaglandins. COX-1 is constitutively expressed in most tissues whereas COX-2 is inducible by inflammation. Naproxen has slightly more selectivity for COX-1 than COX-2.

Pharmacokinetics: Oral bioavailability about 90%. Naproxen is extensively metabolized by liver and about 95% is excreted in the urine. It has a t½ of 12–17 hours. Action lasts for about 10 hours.

Uses:
- First-line drug of alleviating migraine attacks.
- Symptomatic treatment of rheumatoid arthritis (RA), ankylosing spondylitis, and OA.
- Used for fever

Dose: Available as oral suspension and oral tablets. Delayed release formulation use for OA, RA, and ankylosing spondylitis.
- *Pain*:
  - Naproxen conventional tablets—500 mg followed by 500 mg every 12 hours or 250 mg every 6–8 hours.
  - Naproxen sodium conventional tablets—550 mg followed by 550 mg every 12 hours or 275 mg every 6–8 hours.
  - Naproxen sodium extended release tablets—1.1 g once daily. Maximum of 1.65 g for limited period.
- *Use in migraine*: Naproxen sodium 500 mg as single dose (may combine with 85 mg sumatriptan). At least 2 hours between two doses.

Adverse effects:
- Increased risk of cardiovascular events.

- GI ulceration and esophagitis. Concurrent proton pump inhibitor (PPI) use is recommended in those with high risk of GI ulceration, hepatotoxicity, heart failure and edema, hypertension, renal papillary necrosis, and hypersensitivity.

Use in special population:
- Use in pregnancy above 30 weeks may cause premature closure of patent ductus arteriosus and fetal oligohydramnios also has been reported. May cause reversible infertility.
- Secreted in to breast milk. Use with caution.
- <2 years of age-safety is not established.
- Consider lower dosage in hepatic and renal impairment.

NATALIZUMAB

Introduction:
- Humanized immunoglobulin G4 (IgG4) antibody against α4-integrin, a part of VLA4 integrin family
- Indicated in clinically isolated syndrome, relapsing-remitting multiple sclerosis (RRMS) and secondary-progressive multiple sclerosis (SPMS)

Pharmacodynamics: Natalizumab is a monoclonal antibody that binds to α4-integrin (α4-subunit of α4β1 and α4β7 integrins) which is present on cell surfaces of all leukocytes except neutrophils. By doing to, prevents its binding to its receptor, vascular cell adhesion molecule 1 (VCAM-1). Hence, it prevents trafficking of lymphocytes in to the CNS.

Pharmacokinetics: Elimination t½ is approximately 11 ± 4 days in multiple sclerosis. It is dosed every 4 weeks in multiple sclerosis. It is mainly metabolized by endocytosis wherein it is converted to amino acids. Presence of anti-natalizumab antibodies increases its clearance.

Uses:
- Multiple sclerosis
- Crohn's disease

Trials in multiple sclerosis:
- AFFIRM—Natalizumab monotherapy versus placebo (67% risk reduction) in RRMS
- ASCEND—Natalizumab + interferon (IFN) beta (interferon) versus IFN-β + placebo (56% risk reduction) in RRMS
- SENTINEL—42% reduction in disability progression in SPMS

Dose: 300 mg every 4 weeks.

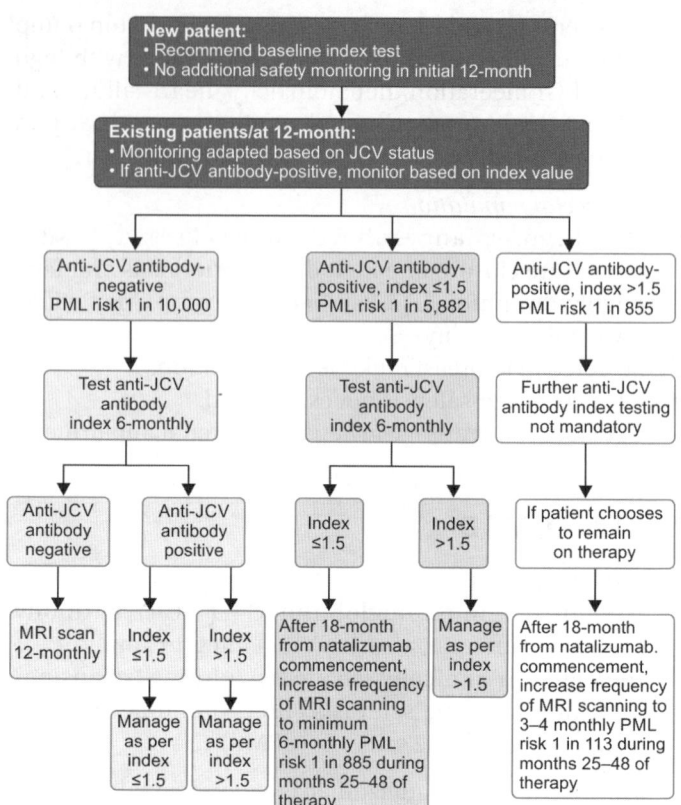

FLOWCHART 1: PML monitoring protocol.

(JCV: John Cunningham virus; PML: progressive multifocal leukoencephalopathy)

Adverse effects:

- Renal or liver impairment can happen within 6 days. Complete blood count (CBC) also needs monitoring.
- Risk of progressive multifocal leukoencephalopathy (PML)

Flowchart 1 uses >2 years or John Cunningham virus (JCV) index > 1.5 poses a high risk of PML.

- There is a risk of rebound relapse after discontinuation.
- Increase risk of other infections such as herpes simplex virus (HSV) and varicella-zoster virus (VZV).

Use in special population and vaccination: It is not recommended in pregnancy and lactation. Killed vaccines can be given while on natalizumab. Live vaccines and live-attenuated vaccines are not indicated while on natalizumab.

NEOSTIGMINE

Introduction: Neostigmine is an reversible inhibitor of acetylcholinesterase (AChE). It is an ionic and water-soluble compound. AChE is an enzyme responsible for breakdown of acetylcholine (ACh) in the synaptic cleft.

Pharmacodynamics: By inhibiting AChE, it enhances neuromuscular transmission and helps in reversal of blockade due to nondepolarizing agents (curare drugs).

Pharmacokinetics: Metabolized by microsomal enzymes of the liver.

Uses:
- Reversal of neuromuscular blockade by nondepolarizing neuromuscular blocking agents—FDA approved.
- Treatment of myasthenia gravis as an add-on to pyridostigmine. Useful especially to improve ptosis in ocular myasthenia.
- Used in intramuscular form for diagnosis of ocular myasthenia gravis.

Dose: 0.03–0.07 mg/kg.

Adverse effects:
- Bradycardia, hypotension, and cardiac arrhythmias
- Can rarely precipitate cholinergic crisis and hypersensitivity

Use in special population: No data is available for pregnancy and lactation. It can be used with caution in liver and renal failure. It can be used with same dose in pediatric and geriatric population.

NICERGOLINE

Introduction: Nicergoline is an ergot alkaloid derivative which became clinically available about 35 years ago in the 1970s. It is used as a vasodilator in cerebrovascular and peripheral vascular disease. It has been used to ameliorate cognitive deficits in vascular dementia.

Pharmacodynamics: It is an alpha-1 antagonist which acts as a vasodilator and improves cerebral blood, also to lungs and the limbs. It also inhibits platelet aggregation.

Uses:
- Cerebrovascular insufficiency, dementia, and peripheral vascular disease

Insufficient data regarding pharmacokinetics and adverse effects.

Dose: 30 mg once or twice daily.

NIMODIPINE

Introduction: Nimodipine is a second-generation 1,4-dihydropyridine calcium channel blocker that was originally approved by the FDA to manage hypertension. Currently, nimodipine is predominantly used to manage vasospasm subsequent to subarachnoid hemorrhage.

Pharmacodynamics: L-type calcium channel blocker and hence prevents depolarization of smooth muscles in the wall of blood vessels. By doing this, nimodipine acts as a vasodilator like any other calcium channel blocker. Nimodipine has selectivity for cerebral vasculature as it is lipophilic and crosses blood brain barrier.

Pharmacokinetics: It has extensive first pass metabolism and hence has decreased oral bioavailability of 13%. Taking with food decreases the plasma concentration. Metabolized by CYP3A4 and CYP3A5 into inactive metabolites, hence interacts with drugs enhancing and inhibiting metabolism of CYP3A4. It has an elimination t½ of 8–9 hours but since the initial elimination is rapid, need frequent dosing every 4 hours.

Uses: Prevention of delayed cerebral ischemia related to spontaneous subarachnoid hemorrhage. No proven role in traumatic subarachnoid hemorrhage.

Off-label uses:
- Assisting recovery after cranial nerve injury
- Migraine prophylaxis
- Ménière's disease

Dose: 60 mg every 4 hours for 21 days in patients with subarachnoid hemorrhage.

Adverse effects:
- Headache, dizziness, nausea, and vomiting
- Case reports of colonic pseudo-obstruction
- IV administration has the US FDA black box warning because it causes bradycardia, hypotension and cardiovascular collapse

Use in special population:
- Dose reduction by 50% needed in patients with cirrhosis
- Formerly category "C" in pregnancy and alternative agents should be preferred
- Not indicated in children

NORTRIPTYLINE

Introduction: Nortriptyline is tricyclic antidepressant which is an FDA approved drug for depression. It inhibits reuptake of serotonin and norepinephrine in to the presynaptic membrane.

Pharmacodynamics: It inhibits reuptake of serotonin and norepinephrine in to the presynaptic membrane. Additionally it inhibits activity of histamine, 5-hydroxytryptamine and acetylcholine. Proposed mechanism in neuropathic pain is increased levels of norepinephrine in the dorsal root ganglia which in turn reduces release of tumor necrosis factor alpha (TNF-α).

Pharmacodynamics: Peak levels attained within 7–8.5 hours but antidepressant efficacy takes 2–3 weeks. Metabolized by CYP2D6 and is excreted via bile.

Uses:
- FDA approved for depression
- Off-label use in neuropathic pain, diabetic neuropathy, migraine prophylaxis, myofascial pain, trigeminal neuralgia, and in smoking cessation

Dose: Started as 12.5 mg and uptitrated. Maximum of 100 mg can be used. It is given as 25 mg three or four times daily.

Adverse effects: Its side effects are mainly due to its anticholinergic action—tachycardia, urinary retention, and xerostomia. It causes QTc prolongation and can cause arrhythmia in toxicity. It has black box warning increase in suicide risk. It can cause drowsiness, gait disturbances and insomnia. Abrupt discontinuation can lead to withdrawal symptoms such as dizziness, nausea, vomiting, headache, and restlessness. Concomitant alcohol usage along with nortriptyline can cause potentiation of effects of alcohol. Usage with monoamine oxidase inhibitors, linezolid, and IV methylene blue can cause serotonin syndrome.

Use in special population: Dose reduction recommended in liver failure. Safety not established in pregnancy and breastfeeding.

NUSINERSEN

Introduction: It is an antisense oligonucleotide (ASO) which promotes the inclusion of exon 7 during SMN2 ribonucleic acid (RNA) splicing. Hence, used in the treatment of spinomuscular atrophy (SMA).

Pharmacodynamics: It is a modified 2'-O-methoxyethyl phosphorothioate ASO that binds to ISS-N1 region in to the intron 7 sequence and blocks access to negative regulators. This binding modulates the splicing of SMN2 messenger RNA (mRNA) transcript, increasing the inclusion of exon 7.

Pharmacokinetics: The drug distributes to CNS and peripheral tissues. The t½ is estimated to be 135–177 days in cerebrospinal fluid (CSF) and 63–87 days in blood plasma. The drug is metabolized via exonuclease (3'- and 5')-mediated hydrolysis and does not interact with CYP450 enzymes. The primary route of elimination is likely by urinary excretion for nusinersen and its metabolites.

Uses and dose:
- Used in SMA
- Route—intrathecal, 12 mg
- Initially four loading doses, first three doses given 15 days apart, fourth dose is given 30 days after the third dose.
- Maintenance dose every 4 months
- General observation is that it is most effective when used in the presymptomatic phase

Adverse effects: Related to intrathecal administration like low pressure headache and pain at the injection site.

Use in special population: Not to be used in pregnancy.

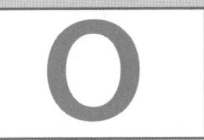

Section Outline

- Olanzapine
- Onasemnogene abeparvovec
- Ondansetron
- Opicapone
- Oxcarbazepine
- Oxybutynin

OLANZAPINE

Introduction: Olanzapine is a second-generation antipsychotic agent which is approved for schizophrenia above the age of 13 years.

Pharmacodynamics: It works by inhibiting D2 (dopaminergic) receptors in the mesolimbic pathway and also 5-HT2A (serotonergic) receptors in the frontal cortex. This effect on serotonergic receptors improves the negative symptoms encounter in schizophrenia such as anhedonia and blunted affect.

Pharmacokinetics: Daily administration leads to steady state levels in 1 week. Has high volume of distribution. Metabolized by CYP1A2 of liver, which is an enzyme prone for polymorphism. Excreted by kidneys with an elimination half-life of 30 hours.

Uses:
- Food and Drug Administration (FDA) approved:
  - Schizophrenia above 13 years of age
  - Bipolar type 1 disorder
  - Combination with fluoxetine (selective serotonin reuptake inhibitor) for treatment of bipolar disorder type 1 and treatment resistant depression. This combination is approved for patients older than 10 years.
  - Approved in combination with samidorphan to attenuate olanzapine-induced weight gain

Dose: Available in oral/intramuscular (IM) forms. Available as 2.5–20 mg tablets.

Adverse effects:
- Weight gain
- Insulin resistance
- Extrapyramidal side effects (lesser than those observed with first generation)
- Use to be avoided in elderly patients with dementia due to higher mortality risk due to cardiac failure and pneumonia
- Low potential for toxicity when used alone

Use in special population: No dose adjustments required in liver and renal failure. Olanzapine may be used for bipolar disorders and schizophrenia in pregnancy, but the clinician needs to carefully evaluate the risk-benefit in consultation with an obstetrician and psychiatrist. Safe in breastfeeding.

ONASEMNOGENE ABEPARVOVEC

Introduction: Onasemnogene abeparvovec is an adeno-associated virus vector-based gene therapy that delivers a fully functional copy of human *SMN* gene into the target motor neuron cells used for spinal muscular atrophy (SMA) approved in 2019.

Pharmacodynamics: Gene replacement which increases the SMN1 copy number.

Uses: Children with SMA < 2 years of age.

Dose: Intravenous (IV) infusion—1.1×10^{14} vector genomes/kg as a single dose. Corticosteroids (prednisolone) at 1 mg/kg should be started 1 day prior to infusion, to be continued for 30 days. This is to prevent liver toxicity. Liver function tests (LFTs) should be repeated after 1 month, if normal steroids may be tapered off over next 28 days. If abnormal, steroids to be continued till transaminases become < 2 ULN, then tapered over 28 days.

Adverse effects: Liver toxicity, immunologic phenomenon (antibody development), and thrombocytopenia.

Use in special population:
- Not to be used in pregnancy.
- Concurrent prednisolone to prevent liver injury as mentioned earlier.

ONDANSETRON

Introduction: It is a very common drug used for vomiting especially chemotherapy-induced vomiting and postoperative vomiting.

Pharmacodynamics: It acts as a selective antagonist at 5-HT3 receptors via central and peripheral mechanisms. Centrally it is present in the area postrema which is the chemoreceptor trigger zone.

Pharmacokinetics: Oral bioavailability is 50–60% but is higher in patients with cancer. Metabolized in the liver by CYP1A2 (main enzyme), CYP2D6, and CYP3A4. Half-life is 3–4 hours. It is excreted by the liver.

Uses:
- FDA approved–prevention of chemotherapy-induced vomiting, postoperative nausea and vomiting (PONV), and radiation-induced nausea and vomiting. It is also used as off-label for nausea and vomiting in pregnancy.
- Also used for alcohol de-addiction
- Cyclical vomiting syndrome in pediatric population. Off-label to treat hallucinations in Parkinson's disease.

Dose:
- Available as oral, IV, or IM forms
- 8 mg oral/IV 12th hourly

Adverse effects:
- Headache, vomiting, and dry mouth
- Insignificant QTc prolongation may occur, especially with IV use. Use of > 16 mg during a single dose is not advised.
- Rarely, Stevens–Johnson syndrome (SJS)

Use in special population:
- No dose modification in mild-to-moderate hepatic failure
- Severe hepatic failure—8 mg maximum per day
- No renal dose modification
- Category B in pregnancy—can be used when other medications do not work
- Exposure to baby during breastfeeding is not significant

OPICAPONE

Introduction: It is a catechol-O-methyltransferase (COMT) inhibitor.

Pharmacodynamics: COMT inhibitors block the peripheral conversion of levodopa to 3-O-methyldopa, increasing both the plasma half-life of levodopa and the fraction of each dose that reaches the central nervous system (CNS).

Pharmacokinetics: Peak plasma concentration is attained in 2 hours. Half-life is 1–2 hours. It is metabolized in liver by sulfation. 70% of drug is excreted in feces via bile.

Uses: Adjunct to carbidopa/levodopa therapy in Parkinson disease patients experiencing frequent "off" episodes.

Dose: 50 mg at bed time.

Adverse effects: Hypotension, hallucination, sleep attacks, dyskinesia, impulse control disorders, constipation, and weight loss.

Use in special population: No dose reduction needed in renal failure of any severity. In mild hepatic impairment, no dose reduction is needed. In moderate hepatic impairment, 25 mg/day is recommended. In severe hepatic impairment, it is best avoided. No adequate data on pregnancy and lactation. Pediatric safety is not established. Do not use concomitantly with nonselective monoamine oxidase (MAO) inhibitors. It is contraindicated in patients with pheochromocytoma.

OXCARBAZEPINE

Introduction: Oxcarbazepine is a 10-keto derivative of carbamazepine which has the FDA approval for treatment of focal seizures in adults and in children above 4 years of age.

Pharmacodynamics:
- Voltage sensitive sodium channel blocker
- Increases potassium conductance
- Modulates high voltage activated calcium channels and prevents glutamate release
- By the earlier mentioned mechanism it inhibits neuronal hyperexcitability

Pharmacokinetics:
- Oral bioavailability—100%
- Metabolized by liver to 10-hydroxycarbazepine which is pharmacologically active, which eventually undergoes glucuronidation.
- Half-life is 2 hours, including that of 10-hydroxycarbazepine—8–15 hours
- Renally excreted
- Drug interaction with phenytoin, phenobarbital, and primidone increases excretion of 10-hydroxycarbazepine and decreases its level.
- 10-hydroxycarbazepine increases level of phenytoin and phenobarbital

Uses: Monotherapy (above 4 years) or adjuvant (above 2 years) for focal seizures with or without secondary generalization.

Dose:
- 600–2,400 mg/day
- Start at low dose and uptitrate—300 mg in two divided doses

Adverse effects:
- Common—somnolence, dizziness, and headache
- Rare—SJS and toxic epidermal necrolysis (TEN). Median time is 19 days.
- Skin rash rate is 5% with oxcarbazepine versus 10–15% with carbamazepine
- HLA-B*1502 is associated with skin rash. Testing for it should be considered before initiating in selected Asian populations (Han Chinese and Thai).
- Hyponatremia
- Agranulocytosis

Use in special population:
- Dose adjustment needed in renal failure. If creatinine clearance (CrCl) < 30 mL/min, start 300 mg/day and titrate slowly
- No specific dose modification is recommended
- Category C, toxicity is usually encountered above 800 mg
- Can continue during breastfeeding with monitoring of infants for adverse effects

OXYBUTYNIN

Introduction: Can be used in pediatric age group >5 years of age.

Pharmacokinetics: It is a selective M3 antagonist, thereby decreases detrusor tone and increases sphincter tone, thereby decreasing urgency.

Pharmacokinetics:
- Bioavailability 6%
- Principally metabolized by CYP3A4
- *Half-life*:
  - Conventional: 2–3 hours
  - Extended release: 2–3 hours
  - Transdermal patch: 7–8 hours

Uses: It is used in overactive bladder. It appears to be as effective as conventional oxybutynin for overactive bladder but less effective than extended release oxybutynin.

Dose in children:
- Conventional (>5 years of age)—5 mg BD
- Extended release preparation (>6 years of age)—5 mg OD

Dose in adults:
- Conventional—5 mg BD or TDS
- Extended release—5 or 10 mg OD
- 1 transdermal system—3.9 mg two times a day twice weekly

Special populations:
- Not studied in renal or liver failure.
- Category B in pregnancy.
- Not studied < 5 years of age

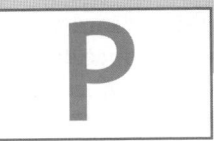

Section Outline

- Paroxetine
- Penicillamine
- Perampanel
- Phenobarbital
- Phenytoin
- Pimavanserin
- Piracetam
- Pitolisant
- Prednisolone
- Pregabalin
- Primidone
- Prochlorperazine
- Procyclidine
- Promethazine
- Propofol
- Propranolol
- Pyridoxine

PAROXETINE

Introduction: It is a selective serotonin reuptake inhibitor.

Pharmacodynamics: Mechanism of action as an antidepressant is linked to potentiation of serotonergic activity in the central nervous system (CNS) resulting from its inhibition of CNS neuronal reuptake of serotonin (5-HT).

Pharmacokinetics: Completely absorbed following oral administration. Widely distributed in the body including CNS and breast milk. More than 93% of the drug is protein bounded. Metabolized by CYP2D6 and eliminated in urine and feces.

Half-life is 21–24 hours.

Uses:
- Major depressive disorder
- Obsessive compulsive disorder
- Panic and anxiety disorder
- Post-traumatic stress disorder

Off-label uses:
- Premenstrual dysphoric disorder
- Premature ejaculation
- Diabetic neuropathy
- Chronic headache

Dose:
Available as oral tablets and suspensions:
- Major depressive disorder—20 mg once daily

- Obsessive compulsive disorder—20 mg once daily
- Panic disorder—10 mg once daily
- Anxiety disorder—20 mg once daily
- Post-traumatic stress disorder—20 mg once daily
- Premenstrual dysphoric disorder—5–30 mg daily
- Premature ejaculation—10–40 mg once daily
- Diabetic neuropathy—40 mg daily
- Chronic headache—10–50 mg daily

Adverse effects:
- *CNS*: Asthenia, somnolence, dizziness, insomnia, tremor, and nervousness
- *Gastrointestinal (GI)*: Nausea, decreased appetite, constipation, and dry mouth
- Impotence, ejaculatory dysfunction, sweating, and anorgasmia in females

Use in special population: In patients with severe hepatic, renal impairment and geriatric/debilitated patients initial dosage of 10 mg or 12.5 mg daily is started. If no clinical improvement is apparent, dosage may be treated with caution up to maximum of 40 mg daily.

PENICILLAMINE

Introduction: It is a conventional disease-modifying antirheumatic drug (DMARD). In neurology, its used as a chelating agent in Wilson's disease.

Pharmacodynamics: Chelate heavy metals such as copper, lead, and mercury and form a soluble complex that is excreted in urine.

Pharmacokinetics: It has a plasma peak time of 1–3 hours and a peak plasma concentration of 1–2 mg/L for the 250 mg dose. The drug's half-life is 4–6 days. More than 80% is protein-bound, and it is excreted in the urine.

Uses:
- FDA approved as a treatment in adults for Wilson disease
- Off-label use for pediatric Wilson disease and lead poisoning

Dose: Available in 250 mg tablets and 125 mg and 250 mg capsules.

Wilson disease:
- *Adult dosing*: 750–1,500 mg/day divided three or four times daily. Dose adjustments are made on the 24-hour urinary copper excretion and free serum copper levels. Dosing to be started slowly, 250 mg OD on alternate days,

then 250 mg OD daily, etc., to the above said maximum dose. Dose to be taken in empty stomach to maximize absorption.
- *Pediatric dosing*: Off-label dosing for pediatric cases of Wilson disease is 20 mg/kg/day divided into 2–3 doses. The maximum dose is 1,000 mg/day.

Lead poisoning: Oral dose is between 1,000 and 1,500 mg daily in divided doses until the urinary lead stabilizes at <0.5 mg/day.

Adverse effects: Diarrhea and dysgeusia are the most common side effects. Skin rash (elastosis perforans serpiginosa), proteinuria, thrombocytopenia, and leukopenia are the less common side effects. Early rash which appears within 6 months, disappears with treatment and may not reoccur when re-challenged at lower dose. Late rash (after 6 months) may re-occur.

Rare adverse effects:
- Local thrombophlebitis and vasculitis
- Anxiety, agitation, dystonia, Guillain–Barré syndrome, myasthenia gravis, and neuropathy
- Agranulocytosis, aplastic anemia, pure red cell aplasia, sideroblastic anemia, positive ANA titer, and thrombotic thrombocytopenic purpura
- Increased serum alkaline phosphatase, hepatic failure, and intrahepatic cholestasis
- Diplopia, optic neuritis, and visual disturbance
- Tinnitus, renal failure, asthma, interstitial pneumonitis, and pulmonary fibrosis
- May trigger lupus like reactions

Use in special population: In pregnancy to treat Wilson, the clinician must weigh the risk versus benefits and limit dosing to 750 mg daily in capsule form and 1,000 mg daily in tablet form. In breastfeeding women avoidance is recommended based on conflicting human data.

PERAMPANEL

Introduction: It is an AMPA receptor antagonist.

Pharmacodynamics: Mechanism of action is by selective and noncompetitive inhibition of AMPA glutamate receptors on postsynaptic neurons, thereby reducing excessive glutamatergic activity and neuronal excitation.

Pharmacokinetics: Completely absorbed following oral administration. Plasma protein binding is 95–96%.

Extensively metabolized in liver, principally by oxidation followed by glucuronidation. Eliminated in urine and feces.

Uses:
- As a monotherapy or adjunctive therapy for partial-onset seizures in adults and adolescents ≥12 years of age.
- Adjunctive therapy for primary generalized tonic–clonic seizures in adults and adolescents ≥12 years of age.
- Off-label usage in the treatment of Lennox–Gastaut syndrome.

Dose:
- *Oral*:
  - Patients not concomitantly receiving CYP3A4 inducer: Initially, 2 mg once daily at bedtime. Increase dosage by increments of 2 mg daily no more frequently than once a week based on clinical response and tolerability. Recommended maintenance dosage is 8–12 mg once daily.
  - Patients concomitantly receiving CYP3A4 inducer: Initially, 4 mg once daily at bedtime. Increase dosage by increments of 2 mg daily no more frequently than once a week based on individual clinical response and tolerability.

Adverse effects:
- Dizziness, somnolence, headache, fatigue, irritability, falls, nausea, weight gain, vertigo, ataxia, gait disturbance, and balance disorder
- It may cause serious behavioral issues especially in the first 6 weeks of therapy.
- Risk of hypersensitivity and drug reaction with eosinophilia and systemic symptoms (DRESS)
- Increased suicidal risk

Use in special population:
- As the half-life of the drug is increased in hepatic impairment patients dosage titration is recommended.
- As the clearance of the drug is decreased in renal impairment patients close monitoring and dosage titration is recommended
- Inadequate data in pregnancy
- No data available for usage in pregnant and breastfeeding mothers. Consider benefits of breastfeeding along with mother's clinical need for the drug and any potential adverse effects on the infant from the drug.
- Safety and efficacy not established in children <12 years of age and in geriatric age group >65 years of age. Gradual dosage titration is recommended in geriatric age group patients.

PHENOBARBITAL

Introduction: Phenobarbital belongs to the barbiturates class of drugs which is mainly used as an antiepileptic.

Pharmacodynamics: Phenobarbital binds to GABA-A receptor subunit. This binding keeps the chloride ion gates open, resulting in a continuous influx of chloride ions into neuronal cells. This leads to hyperpolarization of the cell membrane and raises the action potential threshold.

Pharmacokinetics: Peak plasma concentration ranges from 30 minutes to 1 hour for oral formulations and is around 5 minutes for IV injection. Metabolized by acetylation in the liver. 25–50% of the unchanged drug is excreted in the urine.
Half-life is 53–108 hours.

Uses:
- Management of both generalized and focal seizures (especially in children)
- To treat status epilepticus (2nd line)
- Prophylaxis of febrile seizures
- To manage insomnia and apprehensiveness
- To treat benzodiazepine and alcohol withdrawal
- Neonatal hyperbilirubinemia

Dose:
- Phenobarbital can be administered through various routes, including oral liquid formulation (20 mg/5 mL), oral tablets (15, 16.2, 30, 32.4, 60, 64.8, 97.2, and 100 mg), intramuscular (IM)/intravenous (IV) solution (65 mg/mL, 130 mg/mL). Rectal administration of phenobarbital has a relative bioavailability of up to 90%.
- 15–50 mg 2–3 times daily, 3–5 mg/kg daily
- *In status*: 15–20 mg/kg IV over 20–30 minutes
- To avoid withdrawal symptoms, patients should gradually taper off the medication rather than discontinuing it abruptly.

Adverse effects:
- *Nervous system*: Agitation, somnolence, confusion, CNS depression, hyperkinesia, ataxia, nervousness, nightmares, psychiatric disturbances, cognitive abnormalities, insomnia, anxiety, hallucinations, and dizziness
- *Respiratory*: Apnea and hypoventilation
- *Cardiovascular*: Hypotension, bradycardia, and syncope
- *Gastrointestinal*: Nausea, vomiting, and constipation
- *Dermatologic*: Exfoliative dermatitis, toxic epidermal necrolysis, and rarely, Stevens–Johnson syndrome

Use in special population: As phenobarbital is a potent inducer of cytochrome P450 enzymes, it should be used cautiously in patients with severe hepatic impairment. Used to be avoided in porphyric patients. Approximately 25–50% of phenobarbital is eliminated in the urine, so the drug should be used cautiously in patients with severe renal impairment. Phenobarbital is considered a pregnancy Category D medicine. Barbiturates are reported to cause fetal damage when administered to a pregnant female patient. Caution is advised when using phenobarbital in nursing mothers since the drug is present in breast milk. If infants exhibit excessive drowsiness or poor weight gain, it is recommended to limit or discontinue phenobarbital.

PHENYTOIN

Introduction: Phenytoin is a hydantoin derivative, a first-generation anticonvulsant drug. The FDA approved phenytoin in 1939 for the treatment of epilepsy.

Pharmacodynamics: Phenytoin works by blocking the voltage-dependent membrane sodium channels responsible for increasing the action potential. This action blocks the positive feedback that sustains high-frequency repetitive firing, thus preventing the spread of the seizure focal point.

Pharmacokinetics: In therapeutic doses, phenytoin is absorbed entirely and reaches peak plasma concentration at 1.5–3 hours. Phenytoin is usually 90% bound to plasma proteins (mostly albumin), and only its unbound form is pharmacologically active.

The hepatic P450 enzyme system metabolizes phenytoin to inactive metabolites (predominantly CYP2C9 and CYP2C19) and is an inducer of CYP3A4, which accounts for many of its drug–drug interactions.

Medications that inhibit these enzymes and increase the phenytoin plasma concentrations are the following drugs amiodarone, cimetidine, cotrimoxazole, disulfiram, fluconazole, metronidazole, chloramphenicol, sodium valproate, 5-fluorouracil, and sulfonamides.

Medications that induce the enzyme system to decrease plasma phenytoin concentrations include alcohol, barbiturates, carbamazepine, theophylline, rifampin, and other medications.

1–5% of the drug is excreted in the urine unchanged. At plasma concentrations below 10 mg/L, elimination will follow first-order kinetics; following saturation of the system due to increased drug concentrations, elimination changes to zero-order kinetics.

Uses: Treatment of generalized tonic–clonic seizures, complex partial seizures, status epilepticus, and trigeminal neuralgia. It is considered the drug of choice for post-traumatic and post-neurosurgical seizures. To be avoided in myoclonic seizures.

Dose: Phenytoin is available in oral and parenteral formulations. Intramuscular administration is not recommended due to its erratic absorption and local reaction. Loading dose is 15–20 mg/kg over 30 minutes. The drug is slowly administered intravenously directly into a large central or peripheral vein through an IV catheter less than 20 gauge, not exceeding a rate of 50 mg/min. It causes cardiac dysfunction if administered faster. Maintenance doses should be divided every 6–8 hours. It requires dilution with sodium chloride.

Crystals will form when diluted with a dextrose solution.

Due to its poor solubility, parenteral phenytoin is available in a solution of propylene glycol and alcohol. Fosphenytoin a water-soluble prodrug of phenytoin, devoid of these compounds, which is only available in an injection formulation can be administered intravenously or intramuscularly.

Adverse effects: Rash, sedation, peripheral neuropathy, phenytoin encephalopathy, psychosis, locomotor dysfunction, hyperkinesia, megaloblastic anemia, decreased bone mineral content, Stevens–Johnson syndrome, toxic epidermal necrolysis, immunoglobulin A deficiency, gingival hyperplasia, DRESS syndrome, cardiovascular collapse, hypotension, arrhythmias, hydantoin syndrome in newborns, purple glove syndrome, and hypertrichosis are the adverse effects.

Use in special population: Loading doses not required in liver and renal failure. Lower doses may be required in geriatric patients.

In obese patients, dose as per ideal body weight. Causes fetal harm in pregnancy. In women who are on phenytoin during pregnancy, higher doses may be required due to altered pharmacokinetics.

PIMAVANSERIN

Introduction: It is an atypical antipsychotic agent.

Pharmacodynamics: Mechanism of antipsychotic action is exerted by a combination of inverse agonist and antagonist activity at serotonin type 2A (5-HT2A) receptors, and to a lesser extent at 5-HT2C receptors.

Pharmacokinetics: Bioavailability is >99.7% following oral administration. Plasma protein binding is 95%. Primarily metabolized by CYP3A4/5 and to a lesser extent by CYP2D6, CYP2J2. Eliminated in urine and feces.

Uses: Management of hallucinations and delusions associated with Parkinson's disease psychosis.

Dose: Available in the form of pimavanserin tartrate as oral tablet and capsule. For treating Parkinson's disease psychosis, oral dose of 34 mg once daily without dosage titration is recommended. If used concomitantly with a potent CYP3A4 inhibitor, reduce dosage to 10 mg once daily.
Half-life is 57 hours, and 200 hours for active metabolite.

Adverse effects:
- Peripheral edema and confusional state
- Risk of QT prolongation

Use in special population: No dosage adjustment is required in hepatic, renal impairment patients and geriatric patients. Safety is not established for pediatric usage. No data available for using in pregnant and lactating mothers.

PIRACETAM

Introduction: It is a cyclic derivative of the neurotransmitter GABA.

Pharmacodynamics: It restores cell membrane fluidity that leads to improved neuronal function and circulation. It also modulates cholinergic and glutaminergic transmission, anticonvulsant property, prevents RBC adhesion to endothelium, and enhances neuroplasticity.

Pharmacokinetics: Predominantly excreted by kidneys. Peak concentration occurs in 30 minutes following oral administration. It has got nearly 100% bioavailability. Half-life (t½) in plasma is 5 hours whereas in cerebrospinal fluid (CSF), it is 8 hours.

Uses: Cognitive impairment, vertigo, dyslexia, cortical myoclonus and sickle cell crisis. In cortical myoclonus, it should be used along with other anti-myoclonus therapies.

Dose: For cognitive disorders and vertigo, it is 2.4–4.8 g daily PO, for dyslexia, it is 3.2 g daily PO, for cortical myoclonus, it is 7.2–24.0 g daily PO, for prophylaxis of vaso-occlusive crises in sickle cell anemia, it is 160 mg/kg/day PO, and for remission of vaso-occlusive crises, it is 300 mg/kg/day IV in four divided doses.

Adverse effects: Weight gain, fatigue, depression, and nervousness are some adverse effects.

Use in special population: Drug is contraindicated in end-stage renal disease (ESRD) and dose reduction in renal failure required. It is also contraindicated in pregnancy, lactation, and intracerebral hemorrhage.

PITOLISANT

Introduction: It is selective competitive antagonist and inverse agonist at H3 histamine receptors. It promotes wakefulness.

Pharmacodynamics: By acting as an inverse agonist at the presynaptic H3 receptors, it increases the histamine level and hence promotes wakefulness.

Pharmacokinetics:
- Bioavailability—90%. Peak concentration achieved after a median period of 3.5 hours
- Not affected by food
- Metabolized by CYP2D6
- Half-life is 20 hours

Uses: Narcolepsy.

Dose:
- 17.8–35.6 mg once daily
- Initially 8.9 mg for 1 week followed by 17.8 mg once daily during week 2

Adverse effects:
- Common—insomnia, nausea, and anxiety
- QT prolongation
- Caution when used with drugs that prolong QT interval and CYP2D6 inhibitors

Use in special populations:
- Insufficient data in pregnancy, insufficient data in lactation
- *Hepatic*: Dose adjustment required in moderate-to-severe liver disease
- *Renal*: Dose modification required in moderate-to-severe renal failure
- Safety not established in pediatric age group
- Same dose in geriatric age group

PREDNISOLONE

Introduction: Prednisone is a synthetic glucocorticoid prodrug that is converted by the liver into prednisolone (a beta-hydroxy group instead of the oxo group at position 11), which is the active drug.

Pharmacodynamics: Decreases inflammation via suppression of the migration of polymorphonuclear leukocytes and reversing increased capillary permeability. It also suppresses the immune system by reducing the activity and the volume of the immune system. The antineoplastic effects may correlate with the inhibition of glucose transport, phosphorylation, or induction of cell death in immature lymphocytes. It may have antiemetic effects by blocking the cerebral innervation of the emetic center via inhibition of prostaglandin.

Pharmacokinetics: Half-life is 3.6 hours, excretion by urine.

Use: Bell's palsy, maintenance drug for various autoimmune diseases, demyelinating diseases, meningoencephalitis, some of trigeminal autonomic cephalgias, and DMD.

Dose: 5–60 mg/day PO in single daily dose or divided q6-12 hours.

Adverse effects: The primary adverse effects of prednisone include hyperglycemia, insomnia, increased appetite, hypertension, osteoporosis, edema, adrenal suppression, cataracts, and delayed wound healing, skin fragility, weight gain, increased risk of infections, and fractures. Significant cardiovascular and metabolic effects are hypertension, hyperglycemia, and dyslipidemia.

Use in special population: Amounts of prednisolone in breastmilk are very low. No adverse effects have been reported in breastfed infants with maternal use of any corticosteroid during breastfeeding. It can cause fetal harm, so only can be used if benefit is more than risk.

PREGABALIN

Introduction: It is a structural analog of the inhibitory neurotransmitter gamma-aminobutyric acid (GABA).

Pharmacodynamics: Pregabalin binds to the presynaptic voltage-gated calcium channels (VGCC) at the $\alpha 2\delta$ subunit in the central nervous system and reduces the depolarization-induced calcium influx into neurons, which in turn will decrease the release of excitatory neurotransmitters.

Pharmacokinetics: It is absorbed in the small intestine and proximal colon. Pregabalin controlled release (CR) reaches peak plasma concentrations within 8.0 hours (range: 5.0–12.0), whereas immediate-release pregabalin typically achieves peak concentrations much sooner, around 0.7 hours (range: 0.7–1.5). Pregabalin does not bind to plasma proteins. As the drug is in lipophilic formulation, it readily crosses the blood–brain barrier. Pregabalin is primarily eliminated via renal excretion as an unchanged drug. Mean elimination half-life of pregabalin is 6.3 hours.

Uses: The United States Food and Drug Administration (FDA) approved pregabalin in 2004 for neuropathic pain and seizures.
- Neuropathic pain associated with spinal cord injury
- Neuropathic pain associated with diabetic peripheral neuropathy
- Neuropathic pain originating from postherpetic neuralgia
- Adjunctive treatment for partial-onset seizures in adults with epilepsy
- Treatment of fibromyalgia

Dose: Pregabalin is available in capsule form with strengths of 25, 50, 75, 100, 150, 200, 225, and 300 mg. It is also offered as an oral solution at a concentration of 20 mg/mL, and as extended-release tablets in strengths of 82.5, 165, and 330 mg. When prescribed for the treatment of seizure disorder, pregabalin should be withdrawn gradually to minimize the risk of increased seizure.

Adverse effects: Somnolence and dizziness were the most commonly encountered adverse reactions. Weight gain associated with pregabalin is dose-dependent and occurs in up to 14% of patients receiving 600 mg daily. It also causes angioedema and peripheral edema. FDA Adverse Event Reporting System database reveals that pregabalin has been associated with rhabdomyolysis. Hence, treatment should be discontinued if myopathy is suspected or creatine kinase levels are markedly elevated. Respiratory depression may occur in elderly if used concurrently with other sedatives.

Use in special population:
- It may cause fetal harm in pregnancy. Breastfeeding not recommended while on drug.
- Safety in children <1 month of age is not supported in studies for the management of seizures.
- For other indications, not enough studies in pediatric age group.

- Clearance of pregabalin decreases with age, hence lower doses are to be used in elderly.
- Decreased doses may be needed in patients with renal dysfunction.

PRIMIDONE

Introduction: It is GABAergic drug which metabolized to phenobarbital used in essential tremors.

Pharmacodynamics: The mechanism of action of primidone is not well-known, but it appears to bind centrally with voltage-gated sodium channels and inhibits the monotonous firing of action potentials. Primidone also activates gamma-aminobutyric acid (GABA)-A receptor complex with chloride ionophore, which extends the frequency of opening of the chloride channel, causing hyperpolarization by altering the electrical activity of the nerve cell membrane. The effect of primidone in treating essential tremor is not mediated by the active metabolite PEMA. Because in vivo investigations proved that primidone inhibits TRPM3 and attenuates thermal nociception, this drug could have a role in pain medicine.

Pharmacokinetics: Peak plasma time is 4 hours. Metabolized by liver. Enzyme induced CYP3A4. Elimination half-life is 10–12 hours. Excretion by urine.

Use: FDA-approved indications
- Prophylactic management in seizure, including grand mal, psychomotor, and focal epileptic seizures (not first line choice).

Off-label uses: Essential tremor.

Dose: Seizure disorder—250 mg orally 3 or 4 times daily
- Start 100–125 mg orally at bedtime for 3 days, then 100–125 mg orally twice daily for 3 days, then 100–125 mg orally 3 times daily for 3 days, then 250 mg orally 3 or 4 times daily.
- The maximum daily dose should not exceed 2 g daily.
- Adjust dose based on response and serum levels; gradual dose tapering is necessary to discontinue therapy.

Essential tremor: 50–250 mg orally at bedtime
- Start 12.5–25 mg orally at bedtime for 3 days, then increase by 12.5–25 mg daily or weekly.
- The maximum daily dose should not exceed 750 mg; divide doses >250 mg daily.
- Gradual dose tapering is necessary to discontinue therapy.

Adverse effects: The most common adverse effects of primidone therapy are sedation and drowsiness. Ataxia, diplopia, and nystagmus occur at the initiation of treatment. Other adverse reactions include dizziness, vertigo, epigastric pain, megaloblastic anemia, respiratory depression, polyuria, skin rash, and facial edema.

Use in special population: Primidone is an FDA pregnancy category D drug. There is a risk of infant CNS depression based on limited human data. Dose adjustment needed in renal impairment.

PROCHLORPERAZINE

Introduction: Prochlorperazine is a propylpiperazine-derivative phenothiazine.

Pharmacodynamics:
- Exhibits strong extrapyramidal effects by antagonizing dopamine-mediated neurotransmission at the synapses (by blocking the postsynaptic dopamine receptor sites).
- Exerts antiemetic effect by blocking dopamine receptors in the medullary chemoreceptor trigger zone.
- Sedative effect is exerted by antihistaminic and anticholinergic property.
- It also has weak antagonistic activity against alpha adrenergic and serotonergic receptors.

Pharmacokinetics: Phenothiazines are well absorbed from the GI tract and from *parenteral sites*. High concentration of the drug is distributed into the brain, lungs, liver, kidneys, spleen, and breast milk. It also crosses the placenta. Highly bound to plasma proteins. Principally metabolized in the liver and excreted in urine and feces. Duration of action is 12 hours.

Uses:
- Psychotic disorders—schizophrenia
- Nonpsychotic anxiety
- Nausea and vomiting (migraine, postoperative)

Dose: Available as oral tablets, parenteral injections, rectal suppositories.

Psychotic disorders:
- *Pediatric patients*: 2.5 mg (2 or 3 times). Not exceeding 10 mg on first day. Maximum 20 and 25 mg daily for children 2–5 and 6–12 years of age.
- *Adults*: Oral 10 mg (3–4 times) daily, severely disturbed patients require 100–150 mg daily. IM 10–20 mg for prompt control of symptoms. Can be given every 4–6 hours if prolonged parenteral therapy is needed.

Nausea and vomiting:
- *Pediatric patients*: Children weighing 9–13.2 kg maximum oral dose of 7.5 mg daily is recommended, 13.6–17.7 kg maximum 10 mg daily, 18.2–38.6 kg maximum 15 mg daily dosage is recommended.
- *Adults*: Oral 40 mg daily, IV and IM maximum 40 mg daily, rectal 25 mg twice daily

Nonpsychotic anxiety:
- *Adults*: Oral maximum 20 mg daily (not for >12 weeks)

Adverse effects: Drowsiness, dizziness, amenorrhea, blurred vision, skin reactions, and hypotension are some adverse effects.

Extrapyramidal reactions: Avoid in geriatric patients with underlying dementia, tardive dyskinesia and neuroleptic malignant syndrome.

Use in special population:
- Pregnancy category C
- Use with caution in lactating mothers, hepatic and renal impairment patients
- Lower dosage is recommended in geriatric patients (65 years)
- Avoid usage in children <2 years of age as safety and efficacy are not established in this age group.

PROCYCLIDINE

Introduction: It is a tertiary alcohol and a member of pyrrolidines.

Pharmacodynamics: Nonselective competitive inhibitor of central cholinergic muscarinic receptors (M1, M2, and M4) which crosses blood–brain barrier.

Pharmacokinetics: Elimination half-life is 12 hours. Autonomic effects are maximal within 0.5–2 hours.

Use: Acute dystonias, extrapyramidal symptoms (drug induced), add-on drug for Parkinson disease

Dose: Usually started at 2.5 mg three times a day increasing by 2.5–5 mg/day at interval of 2 or 3 days until optimal response achieved. The usual maintenance dose to achieve response is 15–30 mg/day. For acute dystonias, 5–10 mg IV or IM.

Adverse effects: Agitation, anxiety, blurred vision, cognitive impairment, confusion, constipation, disorientation, dizziness, and tardive dyskinesias

Use in special population: No established studies of its safety in pregnancy and lactation and can be used with caution. Contraindicated in gastrointestinal obstruction, myasthenia gravis, narrow angle glaucoma, and untreated urinary retention.

PROMETHAZINE

Introduction: Tertiary amine that is a substituted phenothiazine.

Pharmacodynamics: Direct antagonist at the mesolimbic dopamine receptors and alpha adrenergic receptors in the brain and exhibits its antihistaminic effects as an H1 receptor blocker.

Pharmacokinetics: Half-life is 10 hours (IM), 9–16 hours (IV), and 16–19 hours (syrup). Metabolized by hepatic enzyme P450 enzyme CYP2D6. 93% protein bound.

Use: Promethazine relieves apprehension, inducing a quiet sleep from which the person can be easily aroused. Other uses are allergy, motion sickness, nausea, vomiting.
It is used in acute dystonia.

Dose:
- Administer 12.5 to 25 mg promethazine orally or rectally at bedtime to provide sedation in children. Adults usually need 25–50 mg before surgery to relieve apprehension and produce quiet sleep for nighttime, obstetrical, or presurgical sedation. Children need 0.5 mg promethazine/pound (body weight) as a preoperative medication combined with adequately reduced narcotic/barbiturate and the required amount of an atropine-like drug.
- The usual recommended adult dosage is 50 mg promethazine with an adequately reduced dose of narcotic/barbiturate and the appropriate dose of a belladonna alkaloid. Postoperative sedation and adjunctive use with analgesic medicines may be achieved by the 12.5–25 mg promethazine in children and 25–50 mg promethazine in adults.

Adverse effects: Sedation, confusion, disorientation, blurring of vision, xerostomia, constipation, may paradoxically causes excitability, restlessness, or rarely seizures. Less common side effects include neuroleptic malignant syndrome, pseudoparkinsonism, acute dystonias, akathisia, and tardive dyskinesias.

Use in special population: Classified as pregnancy category C by the FDA. Little risk to breastfeed infants due to minimal excretion. No dose adjustment needed in renal and hepatic impairment.

PROPOFOL

Introduction: It is an intravenous anesthetic agent prepared in a lipid emulsion which gives its characteristics milky white appearance. The formula contains soybean oil, glycerol, egg lecithin, and a small amount of the preservative EDTA.

Pharmacodynamics: Acts by inhibiting the dissociation of GABA from GABA receptors in the brain and potentiating the inhibitory effects of the neurotransmitter.

Pharmacokinetics: Propofol has a rapid onset of action, which is less than a minute and the duration is approximately 10 minutes. The prolonged or repeated administration will accumulate in peripheral tissues. 97–99% is protein bounded. Metabolized by hepatic oxidation and conjugation to sulfate and glucuronide conjugates. Hepatic clearance is approximately 60%, the remaining 40% via the kidneys.

Uses: Off-label uses—
- Status epilepticus, refractory (children and adults)
- Treatment of refractory postoperative nausea and vomiting

Dose:
- *For sedation-loading*: 5 µg/kg/min (0.3 mg/kg/h over 5 minutes) maintenance—5–50 µg/kg/min (0.3–3 mg/kg/min)
- *IV refractory status epilepticus initial*: 1–2 mg/kg IV injection over 5 minutes, followed by 2–10 mg/kg/h

Adverse effects:
- Transient local pain at the injection site is the most common adverse reaction.
- Hypotension
- Myoclonus
- Occasionally ECG changes (QT interval prolongation)
- Discolored urine (a green tint)
- *Propofol infusion syndrome (PRIS)*: Acute refractory bradycardia, asystole, metabolic acidosis, rhabdomyolysis, hyperlipidemia at rates exceeding 5 mg/kg/h.

Use in special population: Propofol is safe for use in pregnancy but will cross the placenta and may be associated with neonatal CNS and respiratory depression. It is the drug of choice for induction of general anesthesia in pregnancy. No specific renal or liver dosage. Reduced dose in geriatric patients.

PROPRANOLOL

Introduction: It is nonselective beta-adrenergic blocker.

Pharmacodynamics: Beta-blocker, hence has anti-arrhythmic properties. It also has membrane stabilizing property at high doses. In migraine, its precise mechanism is not known but may be attributed to diminishing central catecholaminergic hyperactivity. It also acts beta-adrenergic receptors in the pial vessels.

Pharmacokinetics:
- Complete absorption after oral intake. Absorption increased in children with Down's syndrome
- *Peak effect*: 1-1.5 hours. 100 ng/mL includes adequate beta-blockade
- Crosses blood–brain barrier
- Completely metabolized in the liver
- Half-life is 10 minutes (initial) and 2.3 hours.
- Excreted in feces

Uses: In neurology—
- For prophylaxis of migraine
- Essential tremor

Dose: Start with 80 mg/day. Maximum of 240 mg/day. Response expected within 4-6 weeks in migraine patients.

Adverse effects:
- Adverse effects include nausea, vomiting, sinus bradycardia, heart block greater than first degree, bronchial asthma, and Reynaud's phenomenon.
- Sudden withdrawal may precipitate angina.

Use in special population:
- Use with caution in hepatic and renal dysfunction. Use with caution in geriatric population.
- Category C in pregnancy. Distributed into milk, use with caution
- Same efficacy and safety profile in children

PYRIDOXINE

Introduction: It exists in various forms, including pyridoxine, pyridoxal, and pyridoxamine, which is converted into the active coenzyme pyridoxal 5-phosphate (PLP or P5P) in the body.

Pharmacodynamics: PLP catalyzes various reactions, such as transamination, decarboxylation, racemization, and elimination, in either enzyme-bound or free form. These reactions are significantly facilitated and accelerated in the presence of PLP due to the electron-withdrawing nature of the molecule, which unstabilizes the bonds around the alpha-carbon atom through the system formed with amino acids.

Pharmacokinetics: Half-life is 15–20 days, metabolized by liver to pyridoxal phosphate and pyridoxamine phosphate (active forms).

Use:
- *Nutritional inadequacy*: Pyridoxine hydrochloride is administered through intramuscular or intravenous injections. In cases of nutritional inadequacy, a daily dosage of 10–20 mg of pyridoxine is recommended for 3 weeks. Following this initial treatment, continuing with an oral therapeutic multivitamin preparation containing 2–5 mg of pyridoxine daily for a few weeks is recommended. Alongside these treatments, it is essential to encourage a sufficient and well-balanced diet while addressing any unhealthy eating habits.
- *Pyridoxine/vitamin B6-dependency syndromes*: Specifically, those associated with acute, active seizures may require treatment with pyridoxine (vitamin B6). In such cases, an initial dose of 100 mg of pyridoxine can be administered as a single intravenous (IV) dose. This dose can be repeated at 5–10-minute intervals if necessary. However, the total cumulative dose should not exceed 500 mg.
- *Isoniazid (INH)-induced B6 deficiency*: Total daily dose of 100 mg is recommended for 3 weeks, followed by a daily dose of 30 mg for maintenance.
- *Isoniazid-induced neuropathy prophylaxis*: 25–50 mg orally daily for prophylactic therapy; consider 100 mg by mouth each day in patients with peripheral neuropathy.

Adverse effects: The most well-known adverse effect of vitamin B6 supplementation is sensory neuropathy, but this pathology rarely occurs below toxic doses, which is 1 g/day or more for adults, greater dosages of vitamin B6 below lethal levels may produce indigestion, nausea, breast soreness, photosensitivity, and vesicular dermatoses.

Use in special population: Pregnancy category A drug and safe in lactation.

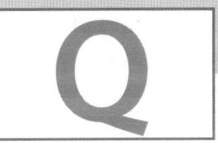

Section Outline

❑ Quetiapine ❑ Quinidine

QUETIAPINE

Introduction: It is a second-generation antipsychotic agent.

Pharmacodynamics:
- Antagonist at 5-HT1A, 5-HT2A, 5-HT2C, and 5-HT6 receptors and at dopamine receptors
- Alpha-1 adrenergic and H1 receptors

Pharmacokinetics:
- Bioavailability is 100%. Affected by food.
- Metabolism—CYP3A4, excretion by urine (major), and feces
- Half-life is 6 hours.

Uses:
- *Food and Drug Administration (FDA) approved*:
  - Symptomatic management of schizophrenia
  - Bipolar disorder—acute manic episodes
- *Non-FDA approved*:
  - Psychosis in patients with Parkinson's disease
  - Insomnia
  - Anxiety disorder
  - For slow channel myasthenic syndrome

Dose:
- *Sedative:* 50–150 mg daily
- *Antidepressant*: 150–300 PO daily
- *For schizophrenia*: Start with 25 mg BD, increase by 25–50 mg. Target 300–400 mg in two or three divided dose by 4th day.
- Mania—100 mg twice daily, increase to 400 mg by 4th day. Maximum 800 mg.

Adverse effects:
- Somnolence, dizziness, dry mouth, constipation, and weight gain
- Increased mortality in geriatric patients with dementia related psychosis

- Worsening of depression and suicidal risk
- Neuroleptic malignant syndrome
- Tardive dyskinesia
- Hyperglycemia
- Possible risk of seizures
- Orthostatic hypotension

Use in special population:
- Pregnancy-category C
- Woman receiving quetiapine should not breastfeed
- Safety and efficacy not established under 18 years
- Dose adjustment required in hepatic conditions but not in renal failure
- May precipitate orthostatic hypotension in elderly

QUINIDINE

Introduction: Quinidine, a stereoisomer of quinine used mainly for management of ventricular arrhythmias and in malaria but used in neurology for management of pseudobulbar affect.

Pharmacodynamics: It is a class 1A antiarrhythmic agent which acts by blocking fast inward current sodium channel. It also has anticholinergic properties.

Pharmacokinetics:
- T_{max}—2 hours. Has high volume of distribution.
- Undergoes hepatic metabolism primarily through hydroxylation mediated by CYP enzymes.
- Major route of elimination is through feces. Only 20% via urine.

Uses:
- *FDA approved for*:
  - *Plasmodium falciparum* malaria
  - Atrial fibrillation
  - Ventricular arrhythmia
  - Pseudobulbar affect—in combination with dextromethorphan

Dose: Fixed dose combination of 10 mg quinidine sulfate with 20 mg dextromethorphan once daily for 7 days. Later may be increased to one capsule every 12 hours.

Adverse effects:
- *Cardiovascular*: QT prolongation
- *Central nervous system (CNS)*: Dizziness, headache, and fatigue
- Skin rash, hepatotoxicity, diarrhea, nausea, esophagitis, and visual disturbances

- Contraindicated in myasthenia
- Can cause hemolysis in glucose-6-phosphate dehydrogenase (G6PD) deficiency. Interaction with CYP enzymes.

Use in special population:
- Dose reduction in hepatic impairment and renal impairment
- Category C in pregnancy. To avoid if possible in nursing woman.
- Safety not established in children
- Safety and efficacy not studied enough in geriatric age group

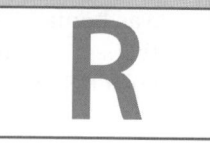

Section Outline

- Ramelteon
- Rasagiline
- Ravulizumab
- Reserpine
- Retigabine
- Riboflavin
- Riluzole
- Risdiplam
- Risperidone
- Rituximab
- Rivaroxaban
- Rivastigmine
- Ropinirole
- Rozanolixizumab
- Rufinamide

RAMELTEON

Introduction:
- Ramelteon is a melatonin receptor agonist used to treat insomnia, particularly for difficulties with sleep onset.
- It mimics the action of melatonin, a natural hormone that regulates the sleep–wake cycle.
- Approved for long-term use due to its favorable safety profile and lack of dependence or withdrawal effects.

Pharmacodynamics:
- Selectively binds to melatonin receptors MT1 and MT2 in the suprachiasmatic nucleus of the brain.
- Promotes sleep by regulating circadian rhythms, particularly influencing sleep onset.
- Does not interact with GABA receptors, avoiding the sedative and dependence effects seen with other sleep medications.

Pharmacokinetics:
- *Absorption*: Rapidly absorbed with peak plasma concentrations within 0.5–1.5 hours after oral administration.
- *Distribution*: Extensively distributed in the body; highly protein-bound (82%).
- *Metabolism*: Undergoes extensive first-pass metabolism in the liver primarily via CYP1A2, with some contribution from CYP2C9 and CYP3A4.
- *Elimination*: Elimination half-life is approximately 1–2.6 hours; excreted mainly in urine as metabolites.

Uses:
- Indicated for the treatment of insomnia characterized by difficulty with sleep onset.
- Not typically used for maintaining sleep or treating middle-of-the-night awakenings.

Dose:
- *Recommended dose*: 8 mg taken 30 minutes before bedtime.
- Should be taken within 30 minutes of going to bed and not administered with or immediately after a high-fat meal, as this can delay its onset of action.

Adverse effects:
- *Common*: Dizziness, fatigue, somnolence, and nausea
- *Rare*: Severe allergic reactions, abnormal thinking or behavior, and depression
- No significant risk of dependence, abuse, or withdrawal symptoms

Use in special population:
- *Elderly*: No dose adjustment required; well-tolerated in elderly patients.
- *Hepatic impairment*: Use with caution in patients with moderate hepatic impairment; contraindicated in severe hepatic impairment.
- *Renal impairment*: No dose adjustment necessary; not significantly affected by renal function.
- *Pregnancy/lactation*: Category C; should be used only if the potential benefit justifies the risk to the fetus, so caution is advised in breastfeeding women.

RASAGILINE

Introduction: Rasagiline is a second-generation, irreversible monoamine oxidase-B (MAO-B) inhibitor used in Parkinson's disease (PD). It enhances dopamine levels by preventing its breakdown, thereby improving motor symptoms like bradykinesia, rigidity, and tremor. As an advancement over selegiline, rasagiline is employed as monotherapy in early PD or as an adjunct to levodopa in advanced PD to manage motor fluctuations, with potential neuroprotective properties.

Pharmacodynamics: Rasagiline selectively inhibits MAO-B, an enzyme that breaks down dopamine in the central nervous system. This inhibition increases dopamine availability in the striatum, alleviating PD motor symptoms. Unlike selegiline, rasagiline does not produce amphetamine-like metabolites, making it better tolerated and safer. It has neuroprotective effects.

Pharmacokinetics:
- *Absorption:* Rapidly absorbed orally with peak plasma concentrations within 0.5–1 hour. Bioavailability is about 36%.
- *Distribution:* Widely distributed, crossing the blood–brain barrier, and binds to plasma proteins (60–70%).
- *Metabolism*: Extensively metabolized in the liver via CYP1A2, producing inactive metabolites like 1-aminoindan.
- *Elimination*: Half-life is approximately 3 hours, with around 60% excreted in urine as metabolites and remainder in feces.

Uses: Rasagiline is primarily used in the management of Parkinson's disease.

It is indicated for:
- Monotherapy in early-stage PD to improve motor function (ADAGIO and TEMPO trials)
- Adjunct therapy to levodopa in patients with advanced PD who experience motor fluctuations, such as "wearing-off" periods.

Dose:
- *Monotherapy*: 1 mg once daily for early-stage PD.
- *Adjunct therapy*: 0.5–1 mg once daily with levodopa for advanced PD to address motor fluctuations.

Adverse effects:
- *Common*: Headache, arthralgia, dyspepsia, depression, dyskinesia, orthostatic hypotension, and nausea
- *Serious but rare*: Serotonin syndrome (with serotonergic drugs) and hypertensive crisis (with excessive tyramine intake)

Use in special population:
- *Elderly*: No dose adjustment needed, but monitor for orthostatic hypotension and falls.
- *Hepatic impairment*: Contraindicated in severe impairment; lower doses for mild-to-moderate impairment.
- *Renal impairment*: No major dose adjustments needed.
- *Pregnancy and lactation*: Use only if benefits outweigh risks; unknown if excreted in milk, so caution is advised.

RAVULIZUMAB

Introduction: It is a humanized monoclonal antibody which is a terminal complement inhibitor, used in myasthenia gravis.

Pharmacodynamics: It prevents cleavage of C5 into C5a and C5b, hence preventing formation of membrane attack complex.

Pharmacokinetics: Bioavailability after subcutaneous injection is 79%, approximately half-life of 50 days after IV and subcutaneous injections.

Uses:
- FDA approved for anti-acetylcholinesterase (anti-AChR) positive myasthenia gravis (CHAMPION-MG)- improved QMG (Quantitative Myasthenia Gravis) score by more than 5 points
- Approved in Europe and Japan for aquaporin 4 antibody positive neuromyelitis optica spectrum disorder (NMOSD) (CHAMPION-NMOSD)
- Paroxysmal nocturnal hemoglobinuria
- Atypical hemolytic uremic syndrome (HUS)

Dose:
- Available as IV and subcutaneous forms
- Weight-based dose

Loading dose:
- 40–60 kg: 2,400 mg IV
- 60–100 kg: 2,700 mg IV
- >100 kg: 3,000 mg IV

Maintenance:
2 weeks after the loading dose:
- 40 to <60 kg: 3,000 mg IV q8 week
- 60 to <100 kg: 3,300 mg IV q8 week
- ≥100 kg: 3,600 mg IV q8 week

Caution and adverse effects:
- Vaccination against *Neisseria meningitidis* mandatory before starting therapy (2 weeks prior)
- Vaccination against pneumococcus is advisable.
- Serious risk of meningococcal and infection with other capsulated organisms

Use in special population: No data in pregnancy and lactation. No data for use in pediatric myasthenia gravis. No special renal or liver dose adjustments necessary.

RESERPINE

Introduction: Reserpine is an alkaloid derived from the *Rauwolfia serpentina* plant, traditionally used in Indian medicine. It irreversibly binds to the vesicular monoamine transporter 2 (VMAT2) in presynaptic nerve terminals, preventing the storage of neurotransmitters like norepinephrine, dopamine, and serotonin in synaptic vesicles. Initially used to treat hypertension and psychosis due to its neurotransmitter-depleting effects. Reserpine is now less commonly used.

Pharmacodynamics: Reserpine acts as a peripheral adrenergic neuron antagonist by depleting tissue stores of catecholamines (norepinephrine, dopamine), leading to lower blood pressure and sedative effects.

Pharmacokinetics:
- *Absorption*: Well absorbed orally with a bioavailability of 30–40%, slow onset of action, often taking days to weeks for full therapeutic effects.
- *Distribution*: Widely distributed throughout the body, including the central nervous system (CNS), with 96% protein binding.
- *Metabolism*: Undergoes extensive hepatic metabolism, producing inactive metabolites such as trimethylbenzoic acid and methyl reserpate.
- *Elimination*: Excreted slowly via urine and feces, with an elimination half-life of 45–168 hours, contributing to its long-lasting effects.

Uses:
- *Hypertension*: Previously a first-line treatment for essential hypertension due to its ability to reduce peripheral vascular resistance.
- *Psychiatric disorders*: Used in managing conditions like schizophrenia for its sedative and antipsychotic properties.
- *Other uses*: In lower doses, it is used to treat mild-to-moderate anxiety.

Dose:
- *Hypertension*: Initial: 0.5 mg daily for 1–2 weeks; maintenance: 0.1–0.25 mg daily. Higher dosages increase the risk of depression and other adverse reactions.
- *Psychiatric disorders*: 0.5 mg daily, titrating between 0.1 and 1 mg based on response.
- *Tardive dyskinesia*: 0.25 mg every 6 hours, increasing by 0.1–0.25 mg to a maximum of 5 mg daily.

Adverse effects:
- *CNS*: Sedation, depression, suicidal tendencies due to serotonin depletion
- *Cardiovascular system (CVS)*: Bradycardia, orthostatic hypotension, nasal congestion
- *Gastrointestinal tract (GIT)*: Increased gastric acid secretion, ulcers, diarrhea, abdominal cramps
- *Others*: Extrapyramidal symptoms like parkinsonism and tardive dyskinesia

Caution: Use with caution in asthma, gallstones, Parkinson's disease, renal impairment, inflammatory bowel disease, or a history of peptic ulcer disease.

Use in special population:
- *Pregnancy and lactation*: Category C drug; use only if benefits outweigh risks. Avoid during breastfeeding.
- *Elderly*: Increased sensitivity to hypotensive and depressive effects; use lower doses with careful monitoring.
- *Pediatrics*: Rarely used due to safer alternatives.

RETIGABINE

Introduction:
- Retigabine (also known as *ezogabine*) is an antiepileptic drug (AED).
- It was used to treat partial-onset seizures in adults.
- Unique mechanism as *a potassium channel opener* (KCNQ/Kv7 channel activator).
- Discontinued in 2017 due to safety concerns, including retinal abnormalities and skin discoloration.

Pharmacodynamics:
- Activates KCNQ2-5 potassium channels, stabilizing the resting membrane potential.
- Reduces neuronal excitability, preventing excessive firing associated with seizures.
- Also enhances GABAergic (inhibitory) neurotransmission.

Pharmacokinetics:
- *Absorption*: Well absorbed orally, with peak plasma levels in 0.5–2 hours.
- *Distribution*: Widely distributed, moderately bound to plasma proteins (80%).
- *Metabolism*: Extensively metabolized in the liver via N-glucuronidation and N-acetylation.
- *Elimination*: Half-life of 6–10 hours; excreted mainly in urine (84%) as metabolites.

Uses:
- Primarily used for adjunctive treatment of focal-onset seizures in adults with epilepsy.
- Discontinued from the market due to safety risks.

Dose:
- *Initial dose*: 100 mg three times daily
- *Maintenance dose*: 200–400 mg three times daily, depending on patient response and tolerance
- *Maximum dose*: 1,200 mg/day

Adverse effects:
- *Common*: Dizziness, somnolence, fatigue, confusion, blurred vision, and urinary retention
- *Serious*: Retinal abnormalities, skin discoloration (blue pigmentation), potential for QT prolongation, and tremor
- Risks led to market withdrawal.

Use in special population:
- *Elderly*: Use with caution; start with lower doses due to increased sensitivity to adverse effects.
- *Hepatic impairment*: Dose adjustment required in moderate-to-severe impairment.
- *Renal impairment*: Dose reduction recommended in patients with significant renal impairment.
- *Pregnancy/lactation*: Limited data; potential risks to fetus. Use only if benefits outweigh risks.

RIBOFLAVIN

Introduction: Riboflavin is vitamin B2 which is used in B2 deficiency and riboflavin transporter defects.

Pharmacodynamics: Converts to coenzymes [flavin mononucleotide (FMN) and flavin adenine dinucleotide (FAD)] which are involved in redox reactions of intermediary metabolism and respiratory chain.

Pharmacokinetics:
- Absorbed from upper gastrointestinal (GI) tract. Food increases absorption.
- Converted to FMN and FAD in the tissues.
- Half-life is 66–84 minutes.

Uses:
- Riboflavin transporter disorders
- Brown–Vialetto–Van Laere syndrome
- Fazio–Londe syndrome
- Migraine prophylaxis

Dose:
- Usual dose in deficiency—3–10 mg/day
- Brown–Vialetto–Van Laere syndrome
- Fazio–Londe syndrome
- 10 mg/kg/day in three divided doses for 1 month. Should increase by 10 mg/kg increments to a maximum dose of 50 mg/kg/day. Some patients may require doses as high as 70 mg/kg.
- Migraine prophylaxis—400 mg daily at least for 3 months.

Adverse effects: It is usually nontoxic.

Use in special population: Category A in pregnancy and category C when used above recommended dietary allowance (RDA).

RILUZOLE

Introduction: It is a glutamate antagonist used to treat amyotrophic lateral sclerosis.

Pharmacodynamics:
The mechanism is largely due to:
- Inhibition of glutamate release and NMDA (N-methyl-D-aspartate) receptors
- Inhibition of intercellular events following excitatory neurotransmission
- Inactivation of voltage-gated sodium channels

Pharmacodynamics:
- Oral bioavailability 60%. Predominantly by CYP1A2 of the liver
- Half-life is 12 hours.

Use: It is FDA approved drug for management of amyotrophic lateral sclerosis. It has shown to improve survival by 2–3 months. It also increases the time to tracheostomy.

Dose: Start at 50 mg OD, the effective dose is 50 mg BD.

Adverse effects:
- Can cause transaminitis which is maximum in the first 3 months. Stop if ALT (alanine aminotransferase) is >5 upper limit of normal.
- Neutropenia

Use in special population:
- No data in pregnancy, lactation, or pediatric age group
- Hepatic—no dose modification, discontinue if ALT > 5 ULN
- No renal dose modification

RISDIPLAM

Introduction:
- Risdiplam is an oral, small-molecule, survival motor neuron 2 (SMN2) splicing modifier.
- Approved for the treatment of spinal muscular atrophy (SMA) in patients of all ages.
- First oral therapy for SMA, offering a noninvasive treatment option.

Pharmacodynamics:
- Increases the production of functional SMN protein by modifying SMN2 pre-mRNA splicing.
- Enhances the inclusion of exon 7, which is crucial for producing stable SMN protein.
- Improves motor function and survival in patients with SMA by addressing the underlying genetic defect.

Pharmacokinetics:
- *Absorption*: Rapidly absorbed with a median time to peak concentration of 1–4 hours.
- *Distribution*: High tissue penetration, crossing the blood–brain barrier; moderate plasma protein binding (~87%).
- *Metabolism*: Extensively metabolized by the liver, primarily via CYP3A.
- *Elimination*: Half-life of approximately 50 hours; excreted primarily in feces (53%), with some renal excretion (28%).

Uses:
- Indicated for the treatment of spinal muscular atrophy (SMA) in pediatric and adult patients.
- Effective across different SMA types (type 1, 2, and 3).

Dose:
- Based on body weight:
  - <20 kg: 0.2 mg/kg once daily
  - ≥20 kg: 5 mg once daily
- Administered orally, can be given with or without food

Adverse effects:
- *Common*: Fever, diarrhea, rash, mouth sores, and joint pain
- *Serious*: Liver enzyme elevations, particularly in the first few months of treatment
- Risk of retinal toxicity observed in animal studies, though not confirmed in humans

Use in special population:
- *Pediatric*: Approved for use in infants 2 months and older; dosing based on body weight
- *Geriatric*: Limited data, but no specific dosage adjustments required
- *Hepatic impairment*: Caution in moderate-to-severe impairment; monitor liver function
- *Renal impairment*: No dose adjustment required for mild-to-moderate impairment; limited data for severe impairment
- *Pregnancy/lactation*: Use only if the potential benefit justifies the risk, so caution is advised.

RISPERIDONE

Introduction: Risperidone is a second-generation (atypical) antipsychotic used in the treatment of schizophrenia, bipolar disorder, and irritability associated with autism. It is recognized for its dual action on dopamine and serotonin receptors, offering a better side effect profile than first-generation antipsychotics.

Pharmacodynamics: Risperidone primarily antagonizes 5-HT2A and D2 receptors, which helps manage both positive and negative symptoms of schizophrenia. It also blocks alpha-1-adrenergic, alpha-2-adrenergic, and histaminergic receptors, contributing to its therapeutic effects and side effects. The antagonism of 5-HT2A receptors reduces the risk of extrapyramidal symptoms (EPS) and improves negative symptoms like social withdrawal.

Pharmacokinetics:
- *Absorption*: Risperidone is well absorbed orally, with peak plasma levels reached within 1–2 hours and a bioavailability of 70%.
- *Distribution*: It is extensively distributed in the body, with around 90% bound to plasma proteins.
- *Metabolism*: It is metabolized in the liver by CYP2D6 to its active metabolite, 9-hydroxyrisperidone (paliperidone).
- *Elimination*: Risperidone and its metabolite are excreted mainly in urine and feces. The elimination half-life ranges from 3 to 20 hours, depending on the metabolic rate.

Uses:
- *Schizophrenia*: Effective for managing both positive and negative symptoms
- *Bipolar disorder*: Used for acute treatment of manic or mixed episodes
- *Autism*: Reduces irritability and aggression in children and adolescents
- *Off-label uses*: OCD, PTSD, and Tourette syndrome

Dose:
- *Schizophrenia*: Start with 1 mg twice daily, increasing to 4–8 mg/day based on response
- *Bipolar mania*: Start with 2–3 mg/day, maintaining at 1–6 mg/day
- *Autism-related irritability*: 0.5–2 mg/day depending on age and response

Adverse effects:
- *Common*: Weight gain, sedation, somnolence, dyspepsia, and constipation

- *Serious*: EPS, hyperprolactinemia, metabolic syndrome, QT prolongation, and falls
- *Rare*: Neuroleptic malignant syndrome (NMS), tardive dyskinesia, urinary retention, precocious puberty, pulmonary embolism, and stroke risk in elderly dementia patients

Use in special population:
- *Pregnancy*: Category C; use if benefits outweigh risks
- *Lactation*: Not recommended due to excretion in breast milk
- *Pediatrics*: Approved for autism-related irritability; careful titration needed
- *Geriatrics*: Lower doses recommended with close monitoring for EPS and cardiovascular risks

RITUXIMAB

Introduction: Rituximab is a chimeric monoclonal IgG1-kappa antibody that targets the CD20 antigen on B lymphocytes. Approved in 1997, it is crucial in managing B-cell non-Hodgkin lymphoma (NHL) and various autoimmune diseases.

Pharmacodynamics: It binds to the CD20 antigen on B cells, leading to their depletion through mechanisms like complement-dependent cytotoxicity (CDC), antibody-dependent cellular cytotoxicity (ADCC), and apoptosis. It selectively targets B cells without affecting stem cells or plasma cells.

Pharmacokinetics: It is administered intravenously with 100% bioavailability. It has a biphasic distribution and is primarily metabolized in the reticuloendothelial system. Its elimination half-life ranges from 18 to 32 days, varying with the disease state and prior doses.

Uses:
- It is FDA approved for treating B-cell NHL, chronic lymphocytic leukemia, rheumatoid arthritis (with methotrexate), granulomatosis with polyangiitis, and microscopic polyangiitis.
- In neurology, it is used in RRMS (relapsing remitting multiple sclerosis), NMOSD, autoimmune encephalitis including anti-NMDAR encephalitis, primary angiitis of CNS, Stiff person syndrome, immune mediated peripheral neuropathies, and myasthenia gravis.

Dose:
- 1 g on day 1 and day 15 or 375 mg/m^2 weekly for 4 weeks
- Give IV methyl prednisolone 100 mg prior to each infusion.

- *Initial infusion*: Start at 50 mg/h, increasing by 50 mg/h every 30 minutes to a maximum of 400 mg/h.
- *Subsequent infusions*: Start at 100 mg/h, increasing by 100 mg/h every 30 minutes.

Retreatment:
- *Option 1*—Uk NMO service practice—monitor CD19 counts monthly. Retreat with 1 g when it rises above 1%
- *Option 2*—Kim et al.—monitor CD19 6th weekly in the 1st year, 8th weekly in the 2nd year and 10th weekly in the 3rd year. Retreat with 375 mg/m^2 when CD19 is >0.05% in the first 2 years and if >0.1% subsequently
- *Option 3*: Repeat single infusions every 6 months

Adverse effects: Contraindications include hypersensitivity to rituximab, active infection like TB, immunocompromised state, severe heart failure, or uncontrolled cardiac disease.

Non-live vaccines should be given 4 weeks prior, live vaccines 8 weeks prior.

Common side effects include infusion reactions (fever, chills), nausea, headache, and hypotension. Severe risks include infections, hepatitis B reactivation, and progressive multifocal leukoencephalopathy (PML). Cardiovascular effects may include PR interval prolongation.

Use in special population:
- *Renal/hepatic impairment*: Use with caution; no specific dose adjustment for renal impairment
- *Pregnancy*: Category C; use if benefits justify risks. Patients can be given 1 g dose 1 month before planned conception
- *Lactation*: With increased risk of relapse of demyelination in the postpartum period, Rituximab may be used during lactation. The levels in breast milk are very low.
- *Geriatric*: Increased risk of infection, careful monitoring required

RIVAROXABAN

Introduction: Rivaroxaban is an oral anticoagulant that selectively inhibits factor Xa, a critical enzyme in the coagulation cascade. It was approved by the FDA in 2011 for the prevention and treatment of thromboembolic events, such as deep vein thrombosis (DVT), pulmonary embolism (PE), and stroke in patients with nonvalvular atrial fibrillation.

Pharmacodynamics: Rivaroxaban inhibits factor Xa, preventing the conversion of prothrombin to thrombin and subsequently inhibiting fibrin clot formation. It acts independently of cofactors like antithrombin III and prolongs prothrombin time (PT), activated partial thromboplastin time (aPTT), and Heptest, providing a predictable anticoagulant effect without routine monitoring.

Pharmacokinetics:
- *Absorption*: Rivaroxaban has an oral bioavailability of 80–100%, with peak plasma concentrations achieved 2–4 hours post-administration. The bioavailability is higher for lower doses and requires food for optimal absorption at higher doses (100% with food).
- *Distribution*: It is 92–95% protein-bound, mainly to albumin, with a volume of distribution of approximately 50 L.
- *Metabolism*: The drug is metabolized by CYP3A4/5 and CYP2J2, and undergoes hydrolysis. It is a substrate for P-glycoprotein (P-gp) and breast cancer resistance protein (BCRP) transporters.
- *Elimination*: The half-life is 5–9 hours in younger individuals, extending to 11–13 hours in the elderly. Rivaroxaban is excreted via urine (36% unchanged) and feces (28% unchanged).

Uses and dosage:
- *Stroke prevention*: In nonvalvular atrial fibrillation (20 mg once daily) (ROCKET AF)
- *Venous thromboembolism (VTE) treatment*: 15 mg twice daily for 21 days, followed by 20 mg once daily
- *Postsurgical prophylaxis*: 10 mg once daily post-hip or knee replacement
- *Coronary artery disease (CAD)/peripheral artery disease (PAD)*: 2.5 mg twice daily plus aspirin for reducing cardiovascular events.

In neurology: Approved for use in CVT as off-label (RESPECT CVT trial, SECRET trial, Action CVT).

Adverse effects:
- *Bleeding*: Ranges from minor bruising to severe gastrointestinal or intracranial hemorrhage.
- *Hepatotoxicity*: Rare but includes elevated liver enzymes and potential hepatic injury.
- *Others*: Includes anemia, dizziness, hypersensitivity reactions, and Stevens–Johnson syndrome.

Reversal of anticoagulation: Andexanet alfa is drug to reverse rivaroxaban activity when there is excessive bleeding or when emergency surgery is to be done. Alternatively use of prothrombin complex concentrates (PCC) at the dose of 25 U/kg or activated prothrombin complex concentrate (aPCC) at the dose of 50 U/kg can be used.

Use in special population:
- *Renal impairment*: Dose adjustment required for moderate impairment; contraindicated in severe cases (CrCl <15 mL/min)
- *Hepatic impairment*: Contraindicated in significant hepatic disease (Child–Pugh B or C)
- *Pregnancy and lactation*: Generally not recommended. Use if benefits justify risks; not recommended during breastfeeding
- *Geriatric*: Careful monitoring due to increased bleeding risk

Discontinuation for surgery or other procedures:
- Stop rivaroxaban at least 24 hours before procedure. For major surgeries, 2 doses have to be skipped.
- Restart rivaroxaban after surgery/procedure as soon as adequate hemostasis is established.

If unable to take oral medication following surgical intervention, consider administering a parenteral drug.

RIVASTIGMINE

Introduction: Rivastigmine is a cholinesterase inhibitor used to treat mild-to-moderate dementia in Alzheimer's and Parkinson's disease. FDA approved in 2000, it is available in oral, transdermal patch, and liquid forms. By enhancing cholinergic function, rivastigmine improves cognitive abilities in affected patients.

Pharmacodynamics: Rivastigmine inhibits acetylcholinesterase (AChE) and butyrylcholinesterase (BuChE), increasing acetylcholine levels in the synaptic cleft. This enhancement of acetylcholine improves neurotransmission in cholinergic neurons, which are deficient in Alzheimer's and Parkinson's-related dementia. Dual inhibition of AChE and BuChE is particularly beneficial in conditions with elevated enzyme levels.

Pharmacokinetics:
- *Absorption*: Rapidly absorbed orally, with peak plasma levels in about an hour and 36% bioavailability after a 3 mg dose. Transdermal administration provides steady plasma concentration.
- *Distribution*: Moderate volume of distribution, indicating wide tissue distribution, including the brain.
- *Metabolism*: Metabolized by cholinesterase-mediated hydrolysis, reducing drug–drug interaction risks.
- *Elimination*: Elimination half-life is approximately 1.5 hours (oral) and 3 hours (patch). Primarily excreted by the kidneys, with <1% unchanged.

Uses:
- *Alzheimer's disease dementia*: Improves cognitive function and delays symptom progression
- *Parkinson's disease dementia*: Manages cognitive symptoms and also improves gait
- *Off-label uses*: Lewy body dementia and other cholinergic deficit conditions

Dose:
- *Oral*: Starts at 1.5 mg twice daily, titrated up to 6 mg twice daily based on tolerance
- *Transdermal patch*: Starts at 4.6 mg/24 hours, increasing to 9.5 mg/24 hours and 13.3 mg/24 hours based on response and tolerance.

Adverse effects:
- *Gastrointestinal*: Nausea, vomiting, diarrhea, and anorexia
- *CNS*: Dizziness, headache, insomnia, and seizures
- *Dermatologic*: Skin reactions with the patch
- *Cardiovascular*: Bradycardia, fainting, and QTc prolongation
- *Hepatobiliary*: Abnormal liver function and hepatitis

Use in special population:
- *Pregnancy*: Category B; use only if clearly needed
- *Lactation*: Not recommended
- *Pediatric*: Not indicated for children
- *Geriatric*: No dose adjustments typically needed

ROPINIROLE

Introduction:
- Ropinirole is a non-ergoline dopamine agonist (D2 receptor agonist)
- Used primarily in the treatment of Parkinson's disease (PD) and restless legs syndrome (RLS)
- Mimics dopamine effects in the brain, improving motor control in PD and reducing symptoms of RLS

Pharmacodynamics:
- Selectively stimulates dopamine D2 and D3 receptors in the brain
- Helps to compensate for the reduced dopamine levels in PD
- Provides symptomatic relief by enhancing motor function

Pharmacokinetics:
- *Absorption*: Well-absorbed orally with peak plasma concentrations in 1–2 hours
- *Distribution*: Widely distributed, crosses the blood–brain barrier, and is ~40% protein-bound
- *Metabolism*: Extensively metabolized by the liver via CYP1A2 to inactive metabolites
- *Elimination*: Half-life of ~6 hours; primarily excreted via urine as metabolites

Uses:
- Treatment of idiopathic Parkinson's disease as monotherapy or adjunct to levodopa
- Management of moderate-to-severe primary RLS

Dose:
- *Parkinson's disease*:
  - *Initial*: 0.25 mg three times daily
  - *Titration*: Increase gradually by 0.25 mg per dose each week
  - *Maintenance*: 0.5 mg to 5 mg three times daily
- *Restless legs syndrome*:
  - *Initial*: 0.25 mg once daily, 1–3 hours before bedtime
  - *Titration*: Gradually increase to a maximum of 4 mg daily

Adverse effects:
- *Common*: Nausea, dizziness, somnolence, orthostatic hypotension, hallucinations, and peripheral edema
- *Serious*: Impulse control disorders (e.g., gambling and hypersexuality), sudden sleep onset, and potential for hypotensive episodes.

Use in special population:
- *Elderly*: Increased sensitivity to adverse effects; careful dose titration recommended
- *Hepatic impairment*: Use with caution; may require dose adjustment due to hepatic metabolism
- *Renal impairment*: No significant adjustment for mild-to-moderate impairment; caution in severe impairment
- *Pregnancy/lactation*: Use during pregnancy only if clearly needed; caution advised during breastfeeding as it may inhibit lactation

ROZANOLIXIZUMAB

Introduction: It is humanized IgG4P monoclonal antibody which is FDA approved for both anti-AChR or muscle-specific kinase (MuSK) positive myasthenia gravis.

Pharmacodynamics: Binds to neonatal Fc leading to decreased levels of circulating IgG antibody.

Pharmacokinetics:
- Has nonlinear kinetics, peak plasma levels are obtained in 2 days
- Metabolized by proteolysis

Uses: FDA approved for both anti-AChR or MuSK positive myasthenia gravis.

Dosing:
- Given by subcutaneous infusion
- <50 kg: 420 mg
- 50 to <100 kg: 560 mg
- >100 kg: 840 mg

Adverse effects:
- Increased risk of infections, aseptic meningitis
- Rarely hypersensitivity reactions

Use in special population: No data in pregnancy, lactation, pediatric age group or in liver and renal failure.

RUFINAMIDE

Introduction: Rufinamide is an antiepileptic drug which is used an adjunctive for seizures in patients with Lennox-Gastaut syndrome (LGS).

Pharmacodynamics: It is a triazole derivative antiepileptic which prolongs inactivated state of voltage-gated sodium channel.

Pharmacokinetics:
- *Bioavailability*: 75–80%
- Undergoes biotransformation in to inactive metabolites by carboxyesters
- Renal excretion
- Half-life is 6–10 hours.

Uses: Adjunctive treatment of seizures in LGS.

Dose:
- Available as oral tablets and suspension (40 mg/mL)
- *Children*: Should be started at 10 mg/kg/day and should be increased by 10 mg/kg on alternate days to a maximum dose of 3,200 mg
- *Adults*: Started at 400–800 mg/day. Maximum of 3,200 mg

Adverse effects:
- Common—headache, nausea, vomiting, and dizziness
- Shortening of QT interval
- DRESS syndrome

Special consideration:
- Hepatic and renal dose modification needed
- Higher doses needed in children because of higher metabolic rate, lower doses in elderly
- Category C in pregnancy

S

Section Outline

- S1P receptor modulators
- Safinamide
- Satralizumab
- Selegiline
- Sertraline
- Sodium oxybate
- Solifenacin
- Sovateltide
- Stiripentol
- Suvorexant

S1P RECEPTOR MODULATORS

Introduction: This group consists of four drugs, i.e., fingolimod, siponimod, ozanimod, and ponesimod. S1P is the most studied lysophospholipid which modulates downstream signaling through a group of G-protein-coupled receptors (GPCRs)-SIPR1–5. They are approved for use in clinically isolated syndrome, relapsing-remitting multiple sclerosis (RRMS), and active secondary progressive multiple sclerosis (SPMS). Ozanimod also been investigated for its use in inflammatory bowel disease.

Pharmacodynamics: Sphingosine-1-phosphate is used by naïve and central memory lymphocytes to exit from the lymph node, hence in its absence gets trapped in the lymph nodes and is cleared. The efficacy is based on the concept of functional antagonism. These drugs act as an agonist at S1P but this leads to internalization of the receptors and hence decreased signaling. Fingolimod is the first approved agent which acts on four of the five S1P receptors, i.e., SIPR1, SIPR3, SIPR4, and SIPR5. Ozanimod is a selective S1P modulator and binds to SIP1R an S1P5R subtypes. Siponimod acts on S1PR1 and S1PR5. Ozanimod also acts on S1PR1 and SIPR5 but affinity for SIPR5 is much weaker. Ponesimod shows high affinity for SIPR1.

Pharmacokinetics: Some S1P modulators are prodrugs that require phosphorylation before showing an affinity for S1P receptors. The pharmacokinetic data, uses, and dosage are summarized in the **Table 1**.

TABLE 1: Pharmacokinetic data, uses, and dosage of S1P modulators.

Drugs	Pharmacokinetics	Pharmaco-dynamics	Dose and use	Side effects	Special populations
Fingolimod	• Prodrug • T_{max}—12–16 hours • CYP3A4 metabolism	SIPR1, SIPR3, SIPR4, and SIPR5	• FREEDOM 1 and 2 trials—relapsing-remitting multiple sclerosis (RRMS) • TRANSFORMS—evaluated against interferon beta-1a in RRMS • Approved in RRMS and pediatric multiple sclerosis (MS)	• First dose cardiovascular toxicity, needs monitoring during first dose. • Common across all drugs—headache, nasopharyngitis, etc. • Reactivation of varicella, cryptococcal infection, macular edema, rare risk of progressive multifocal leukoencephalopathy (PML)	• No dose reduction required but liver function test (LFT) monitoring is required • Safe in renal failure • Unsafe in pregnancy. At least two forms of contraception should be used while taking fingolimod and 2 months after it is stopped • Breastfeeding not recommended while on this medication

Continued

Continued

Drugs	Pharmacokinetics	Pharmaco-dynamics	Dose and use	Side effects	Special populations
Siponimod	• T_{max}—3–4.5 hours • CYP2C9. This has 3 subtypes CP2C9 *1/*3; CP2C9 *2/*3, CP2C9 *3/*3. Its use is contraindicated in the latter as they are slow metabolizers	S1PR1 and SIPR5	• BOLD trial—placebo controlled-RRMS • EXPAND trial-secondary progressive multiple sclerosis (SPMS) • Approved for use in clinically isolated syndrome (CIS), active SPMS, and RRMS	First dose cardiac monitoring required in patients only in patients with preexisting rhythm abnormalities	• LFT monitoring necessary • Not to be used in pregnancy
Ozanimod	• T_{max}—6–8 hours • Metabolized by CYP3A4 and monoamine oxidase B (MAO-B). Hence, concurrent use of MAO-B inhibitors is contraindicated	S1PR1 and SIPR5	Approved for use in RRMS, CIS, and active SPMS (US alone)	No cardiac monitoring required	• Interaction with tyramine containing foods • LFT monitoring
Ponesimod	• T_{max}—2.5–4 hours • Minimal interactions	S1PR1	Use is being studied RRMS	Cardiac monitoring for all patients during first dose	Not enough data

Dosing of siponimod:
- Adults and children >10 years (>40 kg)—0.5 mg OD
- Children/adults <40 kg—0.25 mg OD.
- Use not recommended for use <10 years
- *Multiple sclerosis with CYP2C9 genotypes *1/*1, *1/*2, or *2/*2*:
  - 5-day titration
  - Maintenance dose (day 6): 2 mg/day
  - Titration for the 2 mg/day maintenance dose:
    - Day 1: 0.25 mg (1 × 0.25 mg) PO
    - Day 2: 0.25 mg (1 × 0.25 mg) PO
    - Day 3: 0.50 mg (2 × 0.25 mg) PO
    - Day 4: 0.75 mg (3 × 0.25 mg) PO
    - Day 5: 1.25 mg (5 × 0.25 mg) PO
    - Day 6 and thereafter: 2 mg (1 × 2 mg) PO QD
- *Multiple sclerosis with CYP2C9 genotypes *1/*3 or *2/*3*:
  - 4-day titration
  - Maintenance dose (day 5): 1 mg/day
  - Titration for 1 mg/day maintenance dose:
    - Day 1: 0.25 mg (1 × 0.25 mg) PO
    - Day 2: 0.25 mg (1 × 0.25 mg) PO
    - Day 3 0.50 mg (2 × 0.25 mg) PO
    - Day 4: 0.75 mg (3 × 0.25 mg) PO
    - Day 5 and thereafter: 1 mg (4 × 0.25 mg) PO QD
- *Reinitiation after treatment interruption*: After completing initial titration, if maintenance treatment is interrupted for four or more consecutive daily doses, reinitiate treatment with day 1 of the titration regimen.

SAFINAMIDE

Introduction: Anti-parkinsonian drug—monoamine oxidase B (MAO-B) inhibitor.

Pharmacodynamics: Selectively reversible of MAO-B inhibitor which leads to increased dopamine levels. Has higher selectivity for MAO-B when compared to selegiline and rasagiline. Also blocks activated sodium and calcium channels with inhibition of glutamate release.

Pharmacokinetics: Metabolized in liver, excretion in urine, half-life is 20–26 hours, and only oral form available.

Uses: Parkinson's disease (only as add-on to levodopa/carbidopa), early in the disease as disease-modifying agent but not as good as selegiline or rasagiline for this context. Has antidyskinetic properties.

Dose: 50 mg/day—after 2 weeks, increase to maximum 100 mg/day.

Adverse effects: Hypersensitivity reaction, do not use in severe hepatic impairment, do not use with other MAO inhibitors (worsen hypertension) or SNRI/SSRI (serotonin syndrome). Avoid usage with cheese, can trigger cheese reaction.

Use in special population: Inadequate data about safety in pregnant/lactating women/children <18 years.

SATRALIZUMAB

Introduction: Interleukin-6 (IL-6) inhibitor approved for use in seropositive neuromyelitis optica.

Pharmacodynamics: Humanized monoclonal antibody that targets the (IL-6) receptor. Cytokine IL-6 is thought to be a key cause of neuromyelitis optica spectrum disorder (NMOSD), triggering the inflammation cascade and leading to damage and disability.

Pharmacokinetics: Metabolism not studied. Cleared principally by catabolism. Not eliminated via renal or hepatic pathways. Half-life is 30 days. Only injectable form [subcutaneous (SC)].

As opposed to tocilizumab, satralizumab retains its ability to bind to neonatal Fc receptor which protects it from degradation in the endosomes→re-released in to circulation→binds more IL-6R. This mechanism contributes to its longer half-life.

Uses: NMOSD—aquaporin-4 positive (SAkuraSky and SAkuraStar trials).

Dose:
- *Loading*: 120 mg SC at weeks 0, 2, and every 4 weeks thereafter
- *Maintenance*: 120 mg SC q4 weeks

Adverse effects: Hypersensitivity, hepatitis B/tuberculosis (TB) reactivation, nasopharyngitis, leukopenia, upper, and lower respiratory infections.

Use in special population: Do not use in active TB or active hepatitis B infection. Safety in pregnancy, lactation, and children not established.

SELEGILINE

Introduction: Anti-parkinsonian drug—irreversible selective MAO-B inhibitor.

Pharmacodynamics: Selective MAO-B inhibitor—interferes with dopamine reuptake at synapse.

Pharmacokinetics: Metabolized in liver, excreted in urine, and half-life is 10 hours.

Uses: Parkinson's disease early in the disease as disease modifying agent. It is used as an add-on agent to levodopa for symptomatic management.

Dose: 5 mg OD (maximum 10 mg/day)—use in combination with levodopa/carbidopa. Can taper levodopa by 10–30% after 2–3 days of starting selegiline therapy.

Adverse effects: Hypersensitivity, dyskinesia, trigger mania in bipolar patients, irritation of buccal mucosa, exacerbation of hallucinations/psychosis/compulsive behavior, hypertension, serotonin syndrome, and somnolence.

Use in special population:
- No renal/hepatic dose modification required.
- Not enough information on pregnant/lactating/children.

SERTRALINE

Introduction: It is selective serotonin reuptake inhibitor (SSRI) and antidepressant.

Pharmacodynamics: Serotonin transporter (SERT) inhibitor. It increases concentration of serotonin in synapses as it prevents its reuptake. It does not block alpha-adrenergic, histaminergic, and muscarinic receptors. It also weakly inhibits norepinephrine and dopamine reuptake.

Pharmacokinetics: It undergoes liver metabolism by multiple CYP enzymes to N-desmethylsertraline, a metabolite that is 5–10 times. It is excreted in both urine and feces. Half-life is 25–26 hours.

Dose: 25–50 mg per daily. Weekly increase by 25 mg. Maximum dose is 400 mg/day.

Uses: Major depression, obsessive–compulsive disorder (OCD), panic disorders, post-traumatic stress disorders, and premature ejaculation.

Adverse effects: Initial worsening of depression and suicidal tendency is increased in young adults. Nausea, vomiting, somnolence, insomnia, tremor, and hyperhidrosis are some common adverse effects.

Use in special population: At least 2 weeks must elapse before starting sertraline if patient is already on MAO inhibitor. Safety is not established in pediatric age group <6 years. It belongs to pregnancy category C. Caution warranted during lactation.

SODIUM OXYBATE

Introduction: Sodium salt of gamma hydroxybutyrate, an endogenous compound and metabolite of the neurotransmitter gamma-aminobutyric acid (GABA).

Pharmacodynamics: Interacts with GABA-B receptors at noradrenergic and dopaminergic neurons, as well as at thalamocortical neurons.

Pharmacokinetics:
- Drug interaction with other central nervous system (CNS) depressants (such as amobarbital, chloral hydrate, eszopiclone, and zolpidem) due to additive CNS depression. Use with caution with sodium valproate (it increases levels of sodium oxybate).
- 95% of the drug is metabolized to CO_2 and excreted by lung. <5% excreted in urine.
- Half-life is 0.5–1 hour.
- Only available in oral form.

Uses: Narcolepsy patients with excessive daytime sleepiness (or) cataplexy.

Dose:
- Adults:
  - Initially 4.5 g/night PO; administer as a single bedtime dose.
  - Increase dose by 1.5 g/night at weekly intervals to recommended dosage range of 6–9 g once per night.
- *Children*:
  - <20 kg: Lower starting dosage, weekly dosage increases.
  - 20–30 kg: Initially ≤1 g HS; increase by 0.5 g weekly; do not exceed 3 g/dose
  - 30–45 kg: Initiate at ≤1.5 g HS; increase by 0.5 g weekly; maximum 3.75 g/dose
  - ≥45 kg: Initiate at ≤2.25 g HS; increase by 0.75 g weekly; maximum 4.5 g/dose

Adverse effects:
- Headache
- Nausea
- Dizziness
- Pharyngitis
- Vomiting

Use in special population:
- No renal dose reduction needed.
- 50% reduction needed in hepatic impairment.
- Insufficient information on use during pregnancy and lactation.
- Safety and efficacy not established in children <7 years.

SOLIFENACIN

Introduction: It is selective M3 muscarinic receptor antagonist.

Pharmacodynamics: M3 receptor blockade results in inhibition of acetylcholine release from postganglionic parasympathetic nerve endings thereby increasing bladder capacity, lowering intravesical pressure and reducing the frequency of bladder contractions.

Pharmacokinetics: It undergoes hepatic metabolism and by CYP3A4 and excreted renally. Bioavailability is 90%. It has a short half-life of 45–68 hours.

Uses: Overactive bladder.

Dose: 7.5 mg and 15 mg prolonged release form once daily.

Adverse effects: Dry mouth, abdominal discomfort, constipation, and blurred vision. Confusion and delirium are less as it has got M3 selectivity and spares M1 receptor which are in abundance in CNS.

Use in special population: Category C in pregnant women. Discontinue nursing or drug during lactation. Dose reduction needed in liver dysfunction, severe renal impairment, and geriatric population and if used along with drugs that inhibit CYP3A4.

SOVATELTIDE

Introduction: Neural progenitor stimulation—stroke.

Pharmacodynamics: Highly selective endothelin B receptor agonist that stimulates neural progenitor cells in the brain, promoting neurovascular remodeling by forming new neurons (neurogenesis) and blood vessels (angiogenesis).

Pharmacokinetics: Insufficient data, available only in intravenous (IV) form, can be given up to 24 hours after stroke.

Uses: Approved for treatment in India for acute ischemic stroke, irrespective of whether thrombolysis was done or not.

Dose: Three doses of sovateltide (each dose 0.3 µg/kg) administered as an IV bolus over 1 minute at an interval of 3 ± 1 hour on day 1, day 3, and day 6.

Adverse effects: Insufficient data.

Use in special population: Safety in pregnancy/lactating women is not established.

STIRIPENTOL

Introduction: Anticonvulsant which acts by potentiating GABA-A receptors used as an adjunct in Dravet disease.

Pharmacodynamics: Unknown but believed to act through:
- GABA-A potentiation
- CYP450 inhibition—increases clobazam level, potentiation of effects of clobazam

Pharmacokinetics:
- Metabolized by liver (CYP1A2, CYP2C19, and CYP3A4)
- *Excretion*: Urine
- *Half-life*: 8.5 hours (children); 4.5–13 hours (adults)
- Available in oral form only

Uses: Dravet syndrome—combination with clobazam only. Not used as monotherapy.

Dose: 50 mg/kg/day PO administered in two or three divided doses; not to exceed 3,000 mg/day.

Adverse effects:
- Somnolence
- Decreased appetite and weight
- Ataxia
- Agitation

Use in special population:
- No absolute contraindications
- No adequate data on usage during pregnancy and lactation
- Do not use in children < 6 months

SUVOREXANT

Introduction: It is an orexin receptor antagonist.

Pharmacodynamics: Orexin neuropeptide plays a vital role in maintaining wakefulness. Increased orexin activity is associated with insomnia. This drug blocks orexin receptor competitively and promotes sleep.

Pharmacokinetics: Half-life is 12 hours but prolonged to 19 hours in moderate hepatic dysfunction. It is metabolized predominantly by CYP3A4 and to a lesser extent by CYP2C19. Oral bioavailability is 82%. Peak concentration occurs in 2 hours after oral ingestion. Majority of the drug is excreted in feces (66%). Systemic exposure and peak plasma concentration is higher in obese people [body mass index (BMI) > 30 kg/m^2].

Uses: Suvorexant is used treat insomnia.

Dose: 10 mg is the starting dose. Maximum 20 mg is advised. If moderate, CYP3A4 inhibitor is used concomitantly 5 mg is suggested.

Adverse effects: Somnolence at higher doses is the common side effect. Complex sleep behaviors such as sleep walking, suicidal tendency, and sleep paralysis are also reported.

Use in special population: In mild-to-moderate hepatic impairment and in any degree of renal impairment no dose reduction is needed. It is contraindicated in narcolepsy and patients on strong CYP3A4 inhibitors. No data regarding its use in pregnancy and lactation. Pediatric safety is not established.

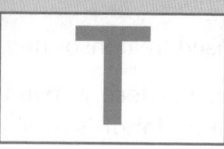

Section Outline

- Tacrolimus
- Tafamidis
- Tapentadol
- Temazepam
- Temozolomide
- Tenecteplase
- Teriflunomide
- Tetrabenazine
- Thalidomide
- Thiamine
- Thiocolchicoside
- Thiopentone
- Tiagabine
- Ticagrelor
- Tizanidine
- Tocilizumab
- Tofersen
- Tolperisone
- Tolterodine
- Tolvaptan
- Topiramate
- Tramadol
- Trientine
- Trihexyphenidyl
- Triptans
- Trospium

TACROLIMUS

Introduction: Calcineurin inhibitor; immunosuppressive agent.

Pharmacodynamics: Tacrolimus suppresses cellular immunity (inhibits T-lymphocyte activation) by binding to an intracellular protein, FKBP-12, and complexes with calcineurin-dependent proteins to inhibit calcineurin phosphatase activity.

Pharmacokinetics: Oral: Incomplete and variable (5–67%); the rate and extent of absorption is decreased (27%) by food (particularly a high-fat meal). Extensively metabolized by the liver via CYP3A4 enzyme. Its half-life is variable: 23–46 hours. Excretion is mainly via feces (93%). Time to peak: Oral: 0.5–6 hours.

Uses:
- *Neurology*: Myasthenia gravis (chronic immunosuppressive therapy)
- *Other*: In organ rejection prophylaxis. Off-label—graft-versus-host disease, intestinal transplant, and pancreas transplant.

Dose: In myasthenia, oral: Initial: 3–5 mg/day or 0.1 mg/kg/day, in one or two divided doses; titrate to achieve target trough concentrations. Typical trough whole blood tacrolimus concentrations should be 10–20 ng/mL in the first month and 5–15 ng/mL after the first month.

Adverse effects: The most common adverse reactions are diarrhea, constipation, nausea, peripheral edema, anemia, infection, tremor, hypertension, and abnormal renal function.

Use in special population: No dosage adjustment is required in kidney disease. In liver impairment, blood concentrations must be closely monitored in Child–Turcotte–Pugh (CTP) C category. In pregnancy, it may cause fetal harm including prematurity, birth defects/congenital anomalies, low birth weight, and fetal distress. In lactation, it is distributed into human milk; effects on infant or milk production unknown. Safety and effectiveness have been established in pediatric liver, kidney, heart, and lung transplant patients.

TAFAMIDIS

Introduction: Benzoxazole derivative; transthyretin (TTR) stabilizer.

Pharmacodynamics: Tafamidis is a TTR stabilizer that selectively binds to TTR at the thyroxine binding sites and stabilizes the tetramer of the TTR transport protein, slowing dissociation into monomers which is the rate-limiting step in the amyloidogenic process.

Pharmacokinetics: Half-life is around 49 hours. Its metabolism is not fully established. Time to peak is around 4 hours. Excretion is mainly through feces (60%).

Uses: In hereditary TTR-mediated amyloidosis and in amyloid cardiomyopathy.

Dose: 61 mg once daily or 80 mg once daily (meglumine form).

Adverse events: In clinical trials, adverse events have been found to be the same as placebo.

Use in special population: No dosage adjustments in manufacturer's labeling for renal or liver disease. Adverse events were found in animal reproductive studies. Data collection to monitor pregnancy and infant outcomes following exposure to tafamidis is ongoing. Breastfeeding is not recommended for mothers on tafamidis.

TAPENTADOL

Introduction: Synthetic, centrally active analgesic; structurally, and pharmacologically related to tramadol.

Pharmacodynamics: Binds to μ-opiate receptors in the central nervous system (CNS) causing inhibition of ascending pain pathways, altering the perception of and response to pain; also inhibits the reuptake of norepinephrine, which also modifies the ascending pain pathway.

Pharmacokinetics: Oral absorption is rapid and complete. It undergoes extensive metabolism, including first pass metabolism; metabolized primarily via phase 2 glucuronidation to glucuronides. The half-life is around 4 hours. It is mainly excreted via urine (99%).

Uses: It is used to manage acute pain and neuropathic pain.

Dose: 50–100 mg every 4–6 hours as needed.

Adverse effects: Nausea, dizziness, vomiting, somnolence, constipation, pruritus, dry mouth, hyperhidrosis, fatigue, headache, vomiting, diarrhea, decreased appetite, anxiety, insomnia, dyspepsia, and hot flush.

Use in special population: In kidney disease, use is not recommended if creatinine clearance (CrCl) < 30 mL/min. A maximum dose of 150 mg per 24 hours is recommended in liver disease. Use is not recommended in CTP class C. No human studies have been done in pregnancy and lactation. Safety and efficacy not established in children <18 years of age.

TEMAZEPAM

Introduction: It is a medication of the benzodiazepine class (short acting).

Pharmacodynamics: It enhances gamma-aminobutyric acid (GABA)-mediated inhibition of synaptic transmission through binding to the GABA-A receptor.

Pharmacokinetics: It has a short half-life of 8–20 hours. Metabolized in liver and excreted through kidneys and has bioavailability of 96%.

Uses: To treat insomnia and anxiety disorders.

Dose: Available in 7.5, 15, 22.5, and 30 mg oral formulations.

Adverse effects: Common side effects include drowsiness, confusion, lethargy, dizziness, and euphoria. Serious side effects include hallucinations, respiratory depression, hypotension, and anaphylaxis.

Use in special population: Use with alcohol and opioids is not recommended, use during pregnancy or breastfeeding is not recommended, in renal failure drug should not be used.

TEMOZOLOMIDE

Introduction: It is an oral alkylating anticancer medication.

Pharmacodynamics: It acts by producing deoxyribonucleic acid (DNA) cross-linkages, thus inhibiting DNA and cellular replication by depositing methyl groups on DNA guanine bases.

Pharmacokinetics: It is excreted by renal excretion. Half-life is 1.8 hours, oral bioavailability is 100%.

Uses: Used in the treatment of brain tumors such as glioblastoma and anaplastic astrocytoma.

Dose: Available in 5, 20, 100, 140, 180, 250 mg oral form, and 100 mg/vial injectable. To administer orally in a single dose on days 1–5 of 28 days cycle for 12 cycles.

Adverse effects: Constipation, anxiety, diarrhea, drowsiness, unusual weight gain, myelosuppression, development of secondary malignancies, pneumococcal pneumonia, hepatotoxicity, and male infertility.

Use in special population: It is approved by the Food and Drug Administration (FDA), need for reduction in dose in renal failure. In pregnancy use, studies are not there. The active alkylating methyl hydrazine is not recovered in urine thus renal function is not expected to affect.

TENECTEPLASE

Introduction: It is a tissue plasminogen activator which is a fibrinolytic agent used as single bolus.

Pharmacodynamics: It is formed by three amino acid substitutions at T, N, and K positions in the native tissue plasminogen activator. This increases the half-life and fibrin selectivity. This also makes it resistant to inhibition by plasminogen activator inhibitor 1 (PAI-1).

Pharmacokinetics: Cleared by the liver. Initial half-life is 20–24 minutes. Terminal half-life is 90–130 minutes.

Uses:
- FDA approved agent for thrombolysis in ST elevation acute myocardial infarction (MI)
- Off-label for thrombolysis in acute ischemic stroke and pulmonary embolism

Dose:
- To be given as intravenous (IV) bolus over 5 seconds.
- MI—0.5 mg/kg
- Stroke—0.25 mg/kg (ATTEST trial)

Adverse effects: Bleeding, anaphylaxis, arrhythmia, and cholesterol embolization. Symptomatic intracranial hemorrhage (ICH) rate is 2.9% when compared to alteplase (2.7%).

Use in special population: Pregnancy—category C. Decision to use in geriatric population, pregnancy, and in patients with severe hepatic dysfunction should be weighed against potential risks. Not indicated in pediatric age group (<18 years).

TERIFLUNOMIDE

Introduction: It is a disease-modifying pyrimidine synthesis inhibitor used in multiple sclerosis.

Pharmacodynamics: It is a dihydroorotate dehydrogenase inhibitor. It is a principle metabolite of leflunomide and hence, decreases the number of activated lymphocytes in the CNS.

Pharmacokinetics: Highly plasma protein bound and undergoes oxidation in the liver. It is mainly eliminated in the feces (37.5%) and urine 22%.

Uses: Oral drug for multiple sclerosis useful in clinically isolated syndrome, relapsing-remitting multiple sclerosis (RRMS) and active secondary progressive multiple sclerosis (SPMS)—TEMSO trial (placebo controlled), TENERE trial (Teriflunomide vs. subcutaneous Interferon beta), and TOWER trial.

Dose:
- Oral form
- 7-14 mg once daily

Adverse effects:
- Contraindicated in patients with severe hepatic dysfunction, pregnancy, or woman planning pregnancy who are not using reliable contraception. Can also cause male infertility. Avoid concomitant leflunomide use or in those with hypersensitivity.

- Not to be used in active tuberculosis (TB)
- Discontinue use if alanine transaminase (ALT) > 3 upper limits of normal (ULN). Also to use concomitant elimination acceleration procedure.
- Accelerated elimination procedure
- Without accelerated elimination, it can take 8 months to 2 years for teriflunomide to be eliminated. This can be done using cholestyramine or activated charcoal.
- Cholestyramine—8 mg PO q8h for 11 days
- Charcoal—50 g BD for 11 days. This eliminates 98% of the drug in 11 days.

Use in special population:
- Avoid in severe liver failure
- No renal dose modification
- Females should use contraception till levels are below <0.02 mg/L.
- Breastfeeding not recommended during use
- Not studied in pediatric/geriatric population (>65 years)

TETRABENAZINE

Introduction: it is a monoamine depletor which acts by inhibiting vesicular monoamine transporter type 2 (VMAT2) inhibitor used to treat tardive dyskinesia and Huntington's chorea.

Pharmacodynamics: A selective VMAT2 inhibitor with little or no affinity toward VMAT1. It has an active metabolite [+]-α-dihydrotetrabenazine ([+]-α-HTBZ) which also binds to VMAT2 with high affinity.

Pharmacokinetics:
- T_{max}—0.5–1 hour. Oxidative metabolism by CYP3A4/5
- Half-life—16–24 hours
- Excretion 60% urine and 30% in feces

Uses: It is used in tardive dyskinesia and Huntington's disease (FDA approved), tic disorders, and Tourette syndrome.

Dose: Started at 12.5 mg, to be titrated to 12.5 mg BD after 1 week. Not to exceed 25 mg in a single dose. In Huntington's disease, maximum dose is 50 mg in poor metabolizers of CYP2D6, 100 mg in extensive CYP2D6 metabolizers. Higher dose up to 200 mg may be used in other movement disorders.

Adverse effects: Somnolence and QTc prolongation are adverse effects. Not to operate heavy machinery when using valbenazine. Baseline electrocardiogram (ECG) is recommended in poor metabolizers of CYP2D6 and

CYP3A4. Suicidal risk (19–35%) and worsening of cognitive decline and parkinsonism in patients with Huntington's disease.

Use in special population:
- No studies in pediatric and geriatric population
- Contraindicated in hepatic impairment
- Pharmacokinetics—not evaluated in renal impairment
- Pregnancy and lactation—limited data

THALIDOMIDE

Introduction: It is a biologic response modifier and has immunomodulatory, anti-inflammatory, antiangiogenic, and sedative and hypnotic activities.

Pharmacodynamics: Thalidomide exhibits immunomodulatory and antiangiogenic characteristics; immunologic effects may vary based on conditions. Other proposed mechanisms of action include suppression of angiogenesis, prevention of free-radical-mediated DNA damage, increased cell-mediated cytotoxic effects, and altered expression of cellular adhesion molecules.

Pharmacokinetics: Metabolism—minimal, half-life—around 5.5 hours, half-life elimination—5.5–7.3 hours, and excretion—urine: 92% and feces <2%.

Uses:
- *Neurology*: Human immunodeficiency virus (HIV) neuropathy.
- *Other*: In multiple myeloma and erythema nodosum leprosum.

Dose:
- Single dose preferably at bedtime varies based on indication
- *For lepra reactions*:
  - Children/adults < 100 kg usually 100 mg daily
  - Children/adults (>12 years)—100–300 mg daily
  - Severe reactions—may go up to 400 mg in divided doses

Adverse effects: Fatigue, hypocalcemia, edema, constipation, sensory or motor neuropathy, dyspnea, muscle weakness, leukopenia, neutropenia, rash/desquamation, weight gain, and thrombosis.

Use in special population: No dosage adjustment required in kidney or liver disease. Use is contraindicated in pregnancy owing to teratogenicity: Amelia, phocomelia, bone defects, ear and eye abnormalities, facial palsy, congenital heart defects, and urinary and genital tract malformations have been reported. Not recommended while breastfeeding.

THIAMINE

Introduction: It is also known as vitamin B1, a water-soluble vitamin.

Pharmacodynamics: Combines with ATP in the liver, kidneys, and leukocytes to produce thiamine diphosphate, which acts as coenzyme in carbohydrate metabolism in transketolation

Pharmacokinetics: It has a short half-life of 14–18 hours and metabolized through phosphorylation.

Uses: It is used in vitamin B1 deficiency and Wernicke's encephalopathy. High dose initially in Wernicke's encephalopathy: 500 mg one to three times a day for 5 days.

Dose: Available in 50 mg, 100 mg, and 250 mg tablet form, 100 mg capsule, and 100 mg/mL parenteral form.

Adverse effects: In very unusual, large doses of thiamine may cause rashes, itching, pulmonary edema, nausea, and hives. Side effects are more common with IV usage compared to oral formulation, drug-drug interactions with loop diuretics and macrolides.

Use in special population: Dextrose should not be administered first in case of thiamine deficiency. Safe for its use in pregnancy and lactation. Stop the drug immediately if adverse effects occur. Coingestion along with loop diuretics is to be avoided.

THIOCOLCHICOSIDE

Introduction: It is a sulfur derivative of colchicoside which is used as muscle relaxant (back spasms).

Pharmacodynamics: Activates GABA-A and hence has muscle relaxant, sedative, and anxiolytic properties. It also has affinity for glycine receptors.

Pharmacokinetics: Bioavailability of 25% after intramuscular use. Metabolized firstly in the liver to an inactive metabolite, then conjugated in the circulation to active metabolite. Half-life is 7.7 hours. Metabolites are mainly found in feces.

Uses: Adjuvants use of painful muscle contractions in adults secondary to underlying spinal pathology.

Dose:
- Oral—4–8 mg BD for 7 days
- Intramuscular—4 mg BD for 5 days

Adverse effects: Sedation, liver injury, allergy, and rhabdomyolysis are the common adverse effects.

Use in special population: Teratogenic—not to be used in pregnancy or lactation. There is insufficient data for its use in renal or liver dysfunction.

THIOPENTONE

Introduction: It is the thiobarbiturate analog of pentobarbital and an analog of thiobarbital.

Pharmacodynamics: It is an ultra-short-acting barbiturate and depressant of the CNS that induces hypnosis and anesthesia, but not analgesia.

Pharmacokinetics: The half-life of the elimination phase after a single IV dose is 3–8 hours. Metabolism is mainly hepatic.

Uses: For the control of convulsive states, as the sole anesthetic agent for brief (15 minutes) procedures, for narcoanalysis and narcosynthesis in psychiatric disorders.

Dose: Anticonvulsant: Adults: 100–250 mg/kg followed by 3–5 mg/kg/min over 15 minutes. Anesthesia, induction: Adults: 3–6 mg/kg; maintenance: 25–100 mg as needed.

Adverse effects: Adverse reactions include respiratory depression, myocardial depression, cardiac arrhythmias, prolonged somnolence and recovery, sneezing, coughing, bronchospasm, laryngospasm, and shivering.

Use in special population: No specific dosage adjustment in kidney or liver disease. Animal or human reproduction studies have not been conducted with thiopentone. Not recommended for breastfeeding mothers.

TIAGABINE

Introduction: It is an anticonvulsant which is useful in focal seizures. It is also useful in panic disorder.

Pharmacodynamics: Inhibits GABA transporter, thereby prevents reuptake of GABA in to the presynaptic terminal.

Pharmacokinetics:
- Bioavailability of about 90%. No relationship with food.
- Principally metabolized by CPY3A4.
- Excreted in feces. Half-life is 7–9 hours.

Uses:
- Adjunctive therapy of focal seizures in adults and children >12 years of age
- Anxiety, neuropathic, and chronic pain

Dose: Start with 4 mg once daily. Maximum dose of 32 mg in two divided doses.

Adverse effects:
- Sedation, dizziness, and depression
- Rarely suicide ideation, hallucination, and delusions

Use in special population:
- No renal dose modification
- Not to be used to in severe liver disease
- In mild-to-moderate liver disease, maintenance dose of 5–10 mg BD should be used.
- Higher doses are required in children and lower in elderly.
- Category C in pregnancy
- Data in lactation limited

TICAGRELOR

Introduction: It is a reversible P2Y12 platelet adenosine diphosphate (ADP) receptor antagonist.

Pharmacodynamics: It is a reversible inhibitor as opposed to clopidogrel or prasugrel. Decrease in cyclic adenosine monophosphate (cAMP) levels leads to decreased exposure of fibrinogen binding sites to glycoprotein (GP) IIb-IIIa and subsequently decreased platelet aggregation.

Pharmacokinetics:
- Bioavailability—36%
- Metabolized by CYP3A4 to active metabolite. Not affected by polymorphism of CYP2C19 unlike clopidogrel
- Fecal excretion
- Half-life—maximum inhibition > 8 hours after the dose. Return to baseline after 5 days

Uses:
- It is used in acute coronary syndrome along with aspirin as an alternative to clopidogrel for 12 months following the event. It is also used in post-coronary artery bypass graft surgery (CABG) patients for 12 months. May be continued beyond 1 year, if tolerated.
- Ischemic stroke
- As an alternative to clopidogrel when resistance is suspected in combination with aspirin in scenarios where dual antiplatelet therapy is indicated [minor

stroke, high risk transient ischemic attack (TIA), and large vessel intracranial atherosclerosis]

Dose:
- Acute coronary syndrome—180 mg loading followed by 90 mg BD for 1 year and 60 mg BD afterward
- Coronary artery disease with no prior MI—60 mg BD
- Stroke—180 mg loading followed by 90 mg BD for 30 days with concomitant aspirin—loading 325 mg, 75–100 mg daily

Adverse effects: Bleeding risk, mild-to-moderate dyspnea, and bradyarrhythmias are common adverse effects.

Use in special population: Avoid use in severe hepatic impairment. No dose modification required in renal failure. Safe in pregnancy. Breastfeeding not recommended during ticagrelor therapy. Not studied enough in pediatric age group to recommend routine use.

TIZANIDINE

Introduction: Centrally acting muscle relaxant which acts as alpha-2 adrenergic agonist.

Pharmacodynamics: Alpha-2 adrenergic agonist, hence has muscle relaxant properties. Has more effect on polysynaptic pathways than monosynaptic pathways. Structurally similar to clonidine but has only fifth to tenth of the antihypertensive property.

Pharmacokinetics:
- Food increases peak plasma concentration. Metabolized by CYP1A2.
- Excreted in the urine
- Half-life is 2.5 hours.

Uses: Management of spasticity in cerebral or spinal injuries, alone or in combination with baclofen.

Dose: Start at 4 mg daily. Maximum of 36 mg in a 24 hours period. The doses can be broken down to three times/day.

Adverse effects: Hypotension, risk of liver injury, sedation, and hallucination are common adverse effects. It can interact with fluvoxamine or ciprofloxacin, both of which increases tizanidine levels.

Use in special population:
- Category C in pregnancy, inadequate data in lactation.
- Safety in pediatric age group not established. Clearance decreased in elderly, hence lower doses to be used.

- Avoid use in severe hepatic failure.
- Use with caution in mild-to-moderate hepatic failure and renal failure.

TOCILIZUMAB

Introduction: It is an immunosuppressive drug, it is a humanized immunoglobulin G1 (IgG1) monoclonal antibody approved by the FDA.

Pharmacodynamics: It selectively binds to interleukin 6 (IL-6) and prevents IL-6 from binding to its receptor on the liver, lung, and synovial fibroblasts.

Pharmacokinetics: Metabolized into smaller proteins and amino acids by proteolytic enzymes via CYP450 system, half-life is 5–13 days, clearance is dose-dependent.

Uses: Severe recurrent anti-myelin oligodendrocyte glycoprotein (MOG)-associated optic neuritis, neuromyelitis optica (both AQP4 positive and negative), rheumatoid arthritis, giant cell arteritis, systemic juvenile idiopathic arthritis, systemic sclerosis, and autoimmune conditions.

Dose: Available as IV and SC routes, usually for adults it is 8 mg/kg once every 4 weeks IV infusion, 162 mg via SC every 3 weeks.

Adverse effects: Allergic reaction, dizziness, melena, hepatic failure, pancreatitis, TB, blurred vision, increased plasma cholesterol, drug–drug interactions with live vaccines, neutropenia, lymphopenia, and TB reactivation.

Use in special population: Avoid using in patients with baseline aspartate transaminase/alanine aminotransferase (AST/ALT) > 10 times the upper normal limit, no adjustment necessary in patients with CrCl > 30, weigh the risk versus benefit in pregnant patients, study on older patients experienced therapeutic improvement similar to younger patients.

TOFERSEN

Introduction: Tofersen is an antisense oligonucleotide indicated in patients with amyotrophic lateral sclerosis (ALS) who harbor SOD1 mutation.

Pharmacodynamics: Antisense oligonucleotide which decreases SOD1 protein levels.

Pharmacokinetics: Directly given to cerebrospinal fluid (CSF). Distributes in to tissues. Undergoes hydrolysis through (3'-5') exonuclease.

Uses: ALS with confirmed SOD1 mutation.

Dose:
- Given via intrathecal injection
- 100 mg per administration (15 mL)
- Loading three doses, 14 days apart. Then maintenance 28 days once thereafter.

Adverse Effects:
- Pain, fatigue, arthralgia, and increased white blood count (WBC) counts
- Aseptic meningitis, myelitis, and radiculitis, papilledema, and raised intracranial tension

Use in special population: No data in pregnancy, lactation, and in pediatric age group. No overall difference in geriatric population.

TOLPERISONE

Introduction: It is a muscle relaxant which is used to relieve spasticity in adults poststroke.

Pharmacodynamics: Centrally acting muscle relaxant. Precise mechanism not elucidated. Postulated to be due to blockage of sodium and calcium channels.

Pharmacokinetics: Inadequate pharmacokinetic data.

Uses:
- Poststroke spasticity
- Cramps
- Neuropathic pain
- Back pain

Dose: 150 mg BD.

Adverse effects: Generally well-tolerated. Risk of anaphylaxis. Headache, nausea, and giddiness.

Use in special population: No sufficient data.

TOLTERODINE

Introduction: It is a medication use in the management of overactive bladder.

Pharmacokinetics: It is a selective M3 antagonist, thereby decreases detrusor tone and increases sphincter tone, thereby decreasing urgency.

Pharmacokinetics:
- Bioavailability—variable (10–76%) and onset of action within 1 hour
- Hepatic metabolism—by CYP2D6 5-hydroxymethyl-tolterodine which is the active metabolite.
- Metabolized by CYP3A4 into inactive metabolites. Renal excretion
- Half-life is 2–2.4 hours for tolterodine and 2.9–3.1 hours for its active metabolite.

Uses: It is used in overactive bladder. It appears to be as effective as conventional oxybutynin for overactive bladder but less effective than extended release oxybutynin.

Dose:
- Conventional—2 mg BD
- Extended release—4 mg OD

Adverse effects: Side effects related to other muscarinic receptor are lower but still reported. Dry mouth, dry eyes, constipation, and tachycardia are common adverse effects.

Use in special population: 50% of the dose in patients with renal and liver dysfunction. No dose adjustments in geriatric population. Efficacy not established <18 years of age. Urinary infections were higher when used in pediatric age group. Category C in pregnancy. Other agents used in overactive bladder.

TOLVAPTAN

Introduction: Selective nonpeptide antagonist of arginine vasopressin V2 receptors.

Pharmacodynamics: By antagonizing the V2 receptors, it increases the free water clearance, thereby increasing sodium levels.

Pharmacodynamics: Bioavailability—40%, CYP3A metabolism, 40% renal excretion, and 59% liver. Half-life is 12 hours.

Uses: Euvolemic and hypervolemic hyponatremia.

Dose:
- 15 mg OD, may increase up to 60 mg OD
- Avoid fluid restriction in the first 24 hours of tolvaptan initiation

Adverse effects:
- Not to be used when rapid increase in sodium levels is needed and in hypovolemic hyponatremia.
- Hepatotoxicity, dehydration, hyperkalemia, and hypernatremia.

Use in special population:
- Avoid use in severe liver and renal failure (CrCl < 10 mL/min).
- Category C in pregnancy. Discontinue drug during lactation. Safety not established in pediatric age group. No dose adjustments in elderly.

TOPIRAMATE

Introduction: It is a second-generation antiepileptic agent approved for use in epilepsy, migraine prophylaxis, and for obesity.

Pharmacodynamics: It acts through multiple channels. It enhances GABA-mediated inhibition, sodium channel blocker, L-type calcium channel blocker, a kainite (type of NMDA receptor) receptor blocker, and also a weak carbonic anhydrase inhibitor.

Pharmacokinetics:
- Oral bioavailability > 80%
- Not affected by food
- 40–50% eliminated unchanged in the absence of other enzyme inducers. No specific CYP isoform has been identified. Those induced by carbamazepine and phenytoin play a role.
- Half-life is 10–15 hours.

Uses:
- Initial monotherapy of focal onset seizures and generalized seizures in adults and children >2 years of age (FDA approved)
- Adjuvant add on therapy for focal onset seizures and generalized seizures in adults and children >2 years (FDA approved)
- Adjunctive treatment of seizures with Lennox–Gastaut syndrome above 2 years of age (FDA approved)
- Adjunctive therapy for Dravet syndrome
- Migraine prophylaxis is adults and adolescents >12 years
- Management of alcohol dependence
- Eating disorder
- Antipsychotic-induced weight gain
- For idiopathic intracranial hypertension (IIH) as an adjuvant to acetazolamide

Dose:
- *Adults*:
  - 200–400 mg/day [without enzyme inducing antiepileptic drugs (AEDs)]
  - 400–600 mg/day (with enzyme inducing AEDs)

- *Pediatric (2-16 years)*:
  - 3 mg/kg/day (monotherapy)
  - 6-9 mg/kg/day (with enzyme inducing AEDs)
- *Migraine*: 25-100 mg/day
- *Alcohol dependence*: 200-300 mg/day

Adverse effects:
- Common—psychomotor slowing, fatigue, impairment of language, weight loss and blurred vision, and suicide ideation
- Life-threatening—metabolic acidosis, oligohydrosis, and hyperthermia
- Rare and nonlife-threatening—bilateral angle closure glaucoma typically reported within 1 month, nephrolithiasis, exaggeration of valproate-induced hyperammonemia

Use in special population:
- No dose modification in liver failure
- 50% dose reduction in those with CrCl < 70 mL/min
- Unsafe in pregnancy and lactation
- Insufficient experience in those >65 years

TRAMADOL

Introduction: It is an opioid agonist.

Pharmacodynamics: It selectively binds to opiate receptors and modulates the inhibition of reuptake of norepinephrine and serotonin through M1 metabolite.

Pharmacokinetics: It is metabolized by CYP2D6 and CYP3A4, bioavailability is 75%, excretion occurs primarily via renal excretion, and half-life is 5-6 hours.

Uses: Used as analgesic in acute pain and chronic cancer pain.

Dose: Available as 50, 100, 200, 300, and 5 mg/mL.

Adverse effects: Nausea, dizziness, pruritus, constipation, vomiting, headache, serious side effects include respiratory depression, adrenal insufficiency, and has drug interactions with CYP2D6 inhibitors.

Use in special population: Approved by FDA, tramadol extended release tablets are not recommended in hepatic impairment, it should be avoided in patients with <30 mL/min CrCl, as tramadol passes through placental barrier not to be given for pregnant patients, it is contraindicated in children <12 years.

TRIENTINE

Introduction: It is a copper-chelating agent and used in Wilson's disease.

Pharmacodynamics: Selective copper-chelating agent which is structurally different from D-penicillamine. Less potent than penicillamine as a copper chelator.

Pharmacokinetics: Highest rate of cupriuresia in the first 4 hours after intake. Food inhibits absorption. Metabolized to 2-acetyl metabolites: MAT and DAT, both of which are weaker chelators. Half-life is 13.8–16.5 hours.

Uses: Alternative as a chelator to D-penicillamine in intolerant patients.

Dose:
- Pediatric patients—trientine hydrochloride—500–750 mg in divided doses. 20 mg/kg/day in two to three divided doses. May increase to 1,500 mg/day in pediatric patients <12 years of age.
- Adults—750–1,250 mg/day, maximum of 2,000 mg in two to four divided doses.
- Trientine tetrahydrochloride—start with 300 mg, titrate to 3,000 mg/day in two divided doses.

Adverse effects:
- Hypersensitivity
- Copper deficiency
- Transient worsening of symptoms

Use in special population:
- No renal and hepatic dose adjustments
- Dosage in pregnancy to be reduced to 25–50% of prepregnancy dosage
- Excreted in breast milk. The American Association for Study of Liver Diseases (AASLD) recommends against their use due to risk of copper deficiency in infant.
- Lower doses may be required in pediatric patients. Not many studies in geriatric patients.

TRIHEXYPHENIDYL

Introduction: It is an anticholinergic agent.

Pharmacodynamics: Acts on parasympathetic nervous system by inhibiting efferent impulses directly, the direct central inhibition of cerebral motor center's occur with high doses, mainly dopamine and M1 muscarinic receptors are affected.

Pharmacokinetics: Metabolized by hydroxylation of the alicyclic groups, elimination half-life is 5–10 hours, absorption from the gastrointestinal tract.

Uses: Tremors, spasms, Parkinson's disease, and dystonia in patients with cerebral palsy.

Dose: Available as 2 mg, 5 mg oral tablets, and as a solution of 2 mg/5 mL.

Adverse effects: Confusion, delirium, constipation, urinary retention, and precipitation of narrow angle glaucoma.

Use in special population: Should not be used in pregnancy, it causes significant congenital disabilities. In older patients, it should be used cautiously due to increased risk of anticholinergic adverse effects, should be used cautiously in patients with renal impairment.

TRIPTANS

- Almotriptan
- Eletriptan
- Frovatriptan
- Naratriptan
- Rizatriptan
- Sumatriptan
- Zolmitriptan

Introduction: It is a selective vascular serotonin type 1 like receptor agonist and 5-HT1 agonist.

Pharmacodynamics: Acts on 5-HT1B/1D receptors and blocks the release of calcitonin gene-related peptide (CGRP) implicated in migraine. Vasoconstriction of cranial vessels via 5-HT1B receptors is another postulated mechanism. Hence, it helps abort acute migraine attack by acting on both vascular and neural targets.

Pharmacokinetics: Metabolized to inactive metabolites primarily by monoamine oxidase (MAO)-mediated oxidative deamination, CYP3A4, and CYP2D6. Half-life is of 3–4 hours and bioavailability is 70%.

Uses: Effective in aborting an acute attack of migraine with or without aura in adults and adolescents aged 12–17 years. It cannot be used for prophylaxis. They can also be used to abort acute attack of cluster headache.

Adverse effects: Nausea, paresthesia, dry mouth, dizziness, and somnolence. Contraindicated in patients on MAO-B inhibitors, selective serotonin reuptake inhibitor (SSRI), serotonin-norepinephrine reuptake inhibitor (SNRI), and ergot as there is a risk of serotonin syndrome. Should not be used in patients with ischemic heart disease, peripheral arterial disease, cerebrovascular syndromes, coronary vasospasm, basilar migraine, and uncontrolled hypertension.

Use in special population: Start at lower dose in geriatric patients. Maximum dosage of 12.5 mg/day is recommended in hepatic and renal impairment. Belongs to category C and should be used in pregnancy only if benefit justifies risk to fetus **(Table 1)**.

TROSPIUM

Introduction: It is another agent which is useful in overactive bladder.

Pharmacodynamics: M3 antagonist which shows good bladder selectivity.

Pharmacokinetics: Bioavailability is 9.6%. High fatty meals reduce absorption and hence should be taken 1 hour before meals. Metabolized by ester hydrolysis. Excreted in feces. Half-life of about 20 hours.

Uses: It is used in overactive bladder. It is as effective as intermediate release preparations of tolterodine and oxybutynin. It is more effective than immediate release tolterodine preparations.

Dose: 20 mg BD.

Adverse effects: Dry mouth, constipation, and rarely angle closure glaucoma.

Use in special population: Pregnancy—category C. Use with caution in lactation. Safety not established in pediatric age group. Use with caution in patients with hepatic impairment. Use a dose of 20 mg OD in patients with renal dysfunction.

TABLE 1: Dosage recommendations for special population.

Drug name	Pharmacokinetics	Route/dose	Remarks
Almotriptan	Metabolized to inactive metabolites primarily by MAO-mediated oxidative deamination, CYP3A4, and CYP2D6. Half-life is of 3–4 hours. 70% bioavailability	6.25 mg or 12.5 mg oral tablet. Dose can be repeated after 2 hours if there is no response. Maximum dose is 25 mg in a 24-hour period	Start at lower dose in geriatric patients. Maximum dosage of 12.5 mg/day is recommended in hepatic and renal impairment. Belongs to category C and should be used in pregnancy only if benefit justifies risk to fetus
Eletriptan	CYP3A4 metabolism. Avoid using the drug within 72 hours of intake of CYP3A4 inhibitor. 50% bioavailability. Half-life is 4 hours. Peak plasma concentration in 1.5–2 hours	Dose 20 mg or 40 mg. If there is no response after 2 hours another dose can be repeated. Do not exceed 80 mg/day	<ul><li>Category C in pregnancy</li><li>Caution advised during lactation</li><li>Contraindicated in severe hepatic impairment</li></ul>
Frovatriptan	<ul><li>Metabolized via CYP1A2 in liver. Peak plasma concentration after 2–4 hours of ingestion. Half-life is 26 hours</li><li>Uses: Acute attack of migraine</li></ul>	Oral formulation. Dose of 2.5 mg. Can be repeated at 2 hour interval. Maximum dose in a single day is 7.5 mg	Slow acting, belongs to category C. Caution while lactating. No dose reduction needed in mild-to-moderate hepatic impairment. Pediatric safety <18 years not established
Naratriptan	<ul><li>Primary hepatic metabolism by a variety of hepatic enzymes</li><li>Half-life is 5–8 hours</li></ul>	1–2.5 mg per oral. Maximum of four doses. Not to exceed 5 mg/day	No sufficient data to support its use in pregnancy
Rizatriptan	Metabolized by monoamine oxidase (MAO)-A. T_{max} is achieved in 1.5 hours. Renally excreted	<ul><li>Available as tablet and films</li><li>Dose: 5–10 mg, not to exceed 30 mg in a day</li></ul>	Fast acting. In US, it is improved for aborting acute migraine attack in patients above age 6 years

Continued

Continued

Drug name	Pharmacokinetics	Route/dose	Remarks
Sumatriptan	• Rapidly absorbed but has only oral bioavailability of 14%. 100% after subcutaneous administration • Metabolized by MOA-A	• Oral: 25 mg, 50 mg, and 100 mg tablet. Available in combination with naproxen (85 mg/500 mg)—more than two doses in 24 hours is not recommended. Maximum 200 mg/day • Nasal: 5 mg, 10 mg, and 20 mg per actuation as nasal spray and 11 mg as nasal powder. Has faster onset of action • Subcutaneous: 3 mg/0.5 mL, 4 mg/0.5 mL, and 6 mg/0.5 mL. The most effective treatment in acute migraine	In mild-to-moderate hepatic impairment, maximum dose permitted is 50 mg. Contraindicated in severe hepatic impairment. No dose adjustments in renal failure. Not recommended for use in pediatric age group
Zolmitriptan	• Oral bioavailability—40% • Nasal—102% • Renal excretion • Half-life is 3 hours	• Oral: 2.5 mg and 5 mg. Maximum—10 mg/day • Nasal: 2.5–5 mg. Not to exceed 10 mg in a day • Oral dissolvable tablet (ODT): Available as 1.25 mg and 2.5 mg preparations	Nasal spray is approved to age groups 12 years and older

Source: (1) Brar Y, Hosseini SA, Saadabadi A. Sumatriptan. Treasure Island (FL): StatPearls Publishing; 2023.
(2) Abram JA, Patel P. Zolmitriptan. Treasure Island (FL): StatPearls Publishing; 2023.

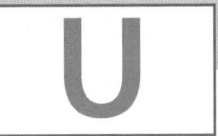

Section Outline

❑ Ublituximab   ❑ Unfractionated heparin

UBLITUXIMAB

Introduction: Novel type 1 chimeric immunoglobulin G1 (IgG1) and glycoengineered anti-CD20 antibody.

Pharmacodynamics: May involve binding to CD20, a cell surface antigen presented to pre-B and mature B lymphocytes results in lysis through mechanism involving antibody-dependent cellular lysis and complement dependent cytolysis.

Pharmacokinetics: Half-life is 22 days. Metabolism is by degradation into small peptides and amino acids by ubiquitous proteolytic enzymes. Administer along with 0.9% NaCl.

Uses: Indicated for treatment of clinically isolated syndrome, relapsing-remitting disease and secondary progressive multiple sclerosis (ULTIMATE I and II).

Dose: First infusion 150 mg intravenous (IV) followed by 450 mg IV after 2 weeks followed by 450 mg IV after 24 weeks of first dose and then for every 24 weeks.

Adverse effects: Infusion reactions (48%), upper respiratory tract infection (URTI) (45%), IgG below lower limits of normal (LLN) at 96 weeks (20.9%). Other minor side effects are lower respiratory tract infection (LRTI), herpes virus infections, and reduced IgG and IgA levels.

Use in special population: There are no studies of its safety in elderly and in patients with renal and hepatic impairment. Do not administer live or live-attenuated vaccines to infants born to mother exposed to ublituximab. Contraindicated in active hepatitis B infection. Chances of progressive multifocal leukoencephalopathy (PML) in human immunodeficiency virus (HIV) infected individuals.

UNFRACTIONATED HEPARIN

Introduction: Glycosaminoglycan found in secretory granules of mast cells. Produced from uridine diphosphate (UDP)-sugar precursors. Mean molecular weight of 15,000 dalton.

Pharmacodynamics: Have no intrinsic anticoagulant activity. It binds to antithrombin and thrombin (larger molecular weight) thus having a quicker onset of action than low-molecular-weight heparin (LMWH). It also accelerates the antithrombin and factor Xa binding. Factor Xa role in clotting mechanism is affected. Inhibiting factor Xa prevents formation of thrombin from prothrombin. Thrombin converts fibrinogen to fibrin to stabilize the clot which is halted by using heparin. Platelet factor 4 in platelet rich thrombi prevents heparin interaction with antithrombin but do not affect LMWH or fondaparinux. Higher doses bind platelets and prolong bleeding time.

Pharmacokinetics: t½ is 1–8 hours (t½ increase with higher doses). Not absorbed in gastrointestinal (GI) tract hence given parenterally. Bioavailability after subcutaneous injection is 30%.

Uses: Apart from treatment of deep vein thrombosis (DVT), pulmonary embolism, and acute coronary syndromes, it is also used prophylactically in critically ill patients to prevent DVT. In acute ischemic stroke, it is not regularly given but in some situations such as cardioembolic strokes, cervical arteries dissection, thrombophilic conditions, stroke prevention in atrial fibrillation, and cerebral venous sinus thrombosis (CVST).

Dose: Only parenteral form. Can be given subcutaneous or IV. 35,000 units in three to four divided doses to produce two to three times prolonged activated partial thromboplastin time (aPTT) (which is therapeutic level).

Adverse effects: Major bleeding, heparin-induced thrombocytopenia (HIT). Protamine is given in a dose of 1mg for every 100 units of heparin. Protamine should be given slow IV and not to exceed 50 mg over 10 minutes. It binds to longer molecules like heparin hence it has only least action on LMWH toxicity and no effect on fondaparinux.

Heparin-induced thrombocytopenia: Decrease in platelets < 1.5 lakh/mm^3 or decrease in 50% from base 5 or more days of starting heparin should lead to suspicion of HIT. HIT can manifest as venous as well as arterial thrombosis resulting in stroke and myocardial infarction. IgG antibodies against platelet factor 4 and heparin complex result in HIT. HIT occurs in 0.5% of patients receiving heparin and incidence is quite rare with LMWH and fondaparinux. In patients requiring anticoagulation nut developed HIT, bivalirudin and new oral anticoagulants (NOACs) can be used. Warfarin should not be used in HIT as it may precipitate limb gangrene and skin necrosis. Osteoporosis over long-term use.

Use in special population: Drugs of choice for anticoagulation during pregnancy. Contraindicated in active bleeding, coagulopathy, recent major surgeries, acute intracranial hemorrhage, and major trauma.

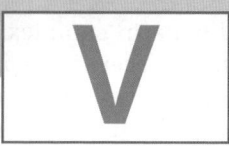

Section Outline

- Valacyclovir
- Valbenazine
- Valproic acid
- Venlafaxine
- Verapamil
- Vigabatrin

VALACYCLOVIR

Introduction: It is a nucleoside analog which is a prodrug of acyclovir.

Pharmacodynamics: Valacyclovir is the L-valine ester of acyclovir which gets converted to acyclovir in the body. Acyclovir is subsequently converted to acyclovir triphosphate. This gets incorporated in to viral deoxyribonucleic acid (DNA) and prevents replication.

Pharmacokinetics: Rapidly metabolized to acyclovir by first pass and hepatic metabolism. Has a bioavailability of 54%. Half-life of 2.5–3.3 hours. Renal clearance.

Uses: It is useful in genital herpes, herpes labialis, and herpes zoster infections. May be used in patients with viral encephalitis (herpes simplex/varicella) when intravenous (IV) acyclovir is not available or when switch over is planned.

Dose: 2 g IV q6–8 hours in patients with herpes simplex encephalitis and 2 g IV q6h in patients with varicella encephalitis. Duration of treatment is a minimum of 10 days.

Adverse effects: Common adverse effects are headache, nausea, and vomiting. It may cause hypersensitivity. It can precipitate in the kidneys and the urinary tract, hence adequate hydration is necessary.

Use in special population: Not indicated in patients with hepatic impairment.

In **Table 1**, patients undergoing hemodialysis—usual dose should be used after the hemodialysis. Category B in pregnancy and can be used while breastfeeding.

TABLE 1: Renal dosing.

Creatinine clearance (mL/min)	Dose
>50	1 g every 12 hours
30–49	1 g every 12 hours
10–29	1 g every 24 hours
<10	500 mg every 24 hours

VALBENAZINE

Introduction: Monoamine depletor which acts by inhibiting vesicular monoamine transporter type 2 (VMAT2) inhibitor used to treat tardive dyskinesia and Huntington's chorea.

Pharmacodynamics: A selective VMAT2 inhibitor with little or no affinity toward VMAT1. It has an active metabolite [+]-α-dihydrotetrabenazine (HTBZ) [+]-α-HTBZ which also binds to VMAT2 with high affinity.

Pharmacokinetics:
- T_{max}: 0.5–1 hour. Oxidative metabolism by CYP3A4/5
- *Half-life*: 15–22 hours
- Excretion 60% urine and 30% in feces

Uses: Tardive dyskinesia (Food and Drug Administration approved) and Huntington's disease (KINECT 2 and KINECT 3 trials).

Dose: Started at 40 mg OD, then increase to 80 mg OD.

Adverse effects: Somnolence and QTc prolongation. Not to operate heavy machinery when using valbenazine. Baseline electrocardiogram (ECG) is recommended in poor metabolizers of CYP2D6 and CYP3A4.

Use in special population:
- No studies in pediatric and geriatric population
- Mild-to-moderate hepatic impairment—40 mg OD maximum
- Mild-to-moderate renal impairment—no dose modification; severe renal failure—not recommended
- Pregnancy and lactation—limited data

VALPROIC ACID

Introduction: Valproic acid (the active moiety), valproate sodium, and divalproex sodium are carboxylic acid-derivative anticonvulsants; also antimanic, other psychotherapeutic, and antimigraine agents. It is an antiepileptic which is considered the drug of choice for generalized seizures in adult males, females of nonreproductive age group, and children with absence seizures when mixed with other seizure types.

Pharmacodynamics: Increase levels of the inhibitory neurotransmitter gamma-aminobutyric acid (GABA) in brain; may enhance or mimic action of GABA at postsynaptic receptor sites; may also inhibit sodium and calcium channels.

Pharmacokinetics:
- No absolute drug interaction contraindications. Use with caution with carbapenems (decreases sodium valproate levels by unknown mechanism) and sodium oxybate (increases sodium oxybate levels).
- *Metabolized by liver—enzymes inhibited*: CYP2C9
- *Excretion*: Urine (30–50%)
- *Half-life*: 7–13 hours (>2 months); 9–16 hours (adults)
- Available in oral/injectable (IV) form (infused over 1 hour—q12h)

Uses:
- Absence seizure—simple and complex. Generally used when present with other seizure types
- Complex partial seizure
- Migraine—prophylaxis
- Bipolar disorder—mania
- Seizures in patients with Dravet syndrome
- Status epilepticus

Dose:
- *Absence seizure/generalized seizures—simple and complex*: 10–15 mg/kg/day (IV or oral)—maximum 60 mg/kg/day
- *Complex partial seizure*: 10–15 mg/kg/day (IV or oral)—maximum 60 mg/kg/day
- *Migraine—prophylaxis*: 500 mg/day—maximum 1,000 mg/day
- *Bipolar disorder—mania*: 750 mg/day—maximum 60 mg/kg/day

Adverse effects:
- Nausea, headache, increased bleeding time, thrombocytopenia, tremor, somnolence, and alopecia
- Can cause polycystic ovary syndrome (PCOS)
- Fatal hepatotoxicity has been reported.
- Life-threatening pancreatitis has been reported.
- Valproate-induced liver failure in patients with mitochondrial disease.

Use in special population:
- Category D in pregnancy. Causes neural tube defects when taken in first trimester of pregnancy.
- Intrauterine exposure can lead to adverse cognitive outcomes and reduces intelligence quotient (IQ) in children.
- No renal dose modification required. No need to decrease dosing in mild-to-moderate liver injury.
- Contraindicated in severe hepatic impairment
- Contraindicated in patients with mitochondrial disease
- Contraindicated in pregnancy—neural tube defects
- Excreted in breast milk
- Use with caution during lactation—need to monitor infant for liver injury

Divalproex sodium is a compound of sodium valproate and valproic acid. Started as 250 mg which is equivalent to 200 mg of sodium valproate.

VENLAFAXINE

Introduction: It is a bicyclic phenylethylamine derivative.

Pharmacodynamics: Bicyclic antidepressant structurally unrelated to selective serotonin reuptake inhibitors (SSRIs), monoamine oxidase inhibitors (MAOIs), and tricyclic antidepressants (TCAs) but it and its metabolite are potent inhibitors of serotonin and nor epinephrine reuptake and weak inhibitors of dopamine reuptake.

Pharmacokinetics: Half-life of 5–11 hours, bioavailability 45%, metabolized in liver by CYP2D6 and excretion in urine, not dialyzable.

Use: Neuropathic pain off-label and migraine prevention off-label.

Dose: 75–225 mg/day PO, onset of relief starts in 1–2 weeks or take up to 6 weeks for full benefit.

Adverse effects: Headache, nausea, insomnia, asthenia, dizziness, dry mouth, ejaculation disorder, and other minor effects are weight loss, abnormal vision, and hypertension.

Use in special population: No established data on malformations in pregnancy but associated with increased risk of preeclampsia and postpartum hemorrhage, relapse of major depression if discontinued during pregnancy. It can be used during lactation. Dose reduction should be done in renal and hepatic impairment (reduce TTD by 50% or more).

VERAPAMIL

Introduction: Papaverine-derived nondihydropyridine calcium channel blocker.

Pharmacodynamics: It inhibits transmembrane influx of extracellular calcium ions across membranes of myocardial cells and vascular smooth muscle cells without change in serum calcium concentration and therefore dilates the coronary and systemic arteries.

Pharmacokinetics: Both IV and PO. Onset PO 1–2 hours, IV 1–5 minutes. Half-life is 4.4–6.9 hours with single dose; 3–7 hours with multiple doses. Metabolism is by hepatic P450 enzyme CYP3A4. Excretion is by urine and feces.

Uses: Prophylaxis of migraine with aura, trigeminal autonomic cephalgias like paroxysmal hemicrania, short-lasting unilateral neuralgiform headache with conjunctival injection and tearing (SUNCT), episodic, and chronic cluster headaches.

Dose: Usual dose is 160–240 mg daily in two to three divided doses and can be increase 80 mg every week up to 480 mg daily. Higher doses can be used in cluster headache. Maximum daily dose should not exceed 1,200 mg.

Adverse effects: Headache and gingival hyperplasia. Less common are constipation, dizziness, hypotension, edema, and rash. It should not be used with beta blockers as they can exaggerate the resulting bradycardia.

Use in special population: Pregnant category C drug. Distributed in milk in minor amounts, discontinue nursing or the drug. In renal impairment, use with caution and monitor ECG. If creatinine clearance (CrCl) < 10 mL/min reduce dose by 25–50%. In cirrhosis, reduce dose by 20–50%.

VIGABATRIN

Introduction: Synthetic derivative of GABA.

Pharmacodynamics: Irreversible inhibitor of GABA transaminases, thereby increasing level of inhibitory neurotransmitter GABA within brain.

Pharmacokinetics: Half-life 5–7 hours in infants, 5–8 hours in young adults, 7.5 hours in adults, 12–14 hours in geriatric patients. Peak plasma time 2.5 hours, protein bound negligible, and excretion 95% in urine.

Uses: Refractory simple and complex partial seizures and infantile spasms.

Dose: 500 mg PO q12h initially then increase by 500 mg every week to target dose of 1.5 g q12h.

Adverse effects: Weight gain (47%), permanent bilateral concentric visual field constriction (30%), fatigue, somnolence, headache, weight gain, and less common are nasopharyngitis, upper respiratory tract infection (URTI), and depression.

Use in special population: Should be used in pregnancy only benefit outweighs the risk, no data available for safety in pregnancy, excreted in breast milk so caution should be taken. Dose adjustment should be done in renal impairment.

Z

Section Outline

- Z-drugs (zolpidem, zaleplon, and zopiclone)
- Zilucoplan
- Zinc acetate
- Zonisamide

Z-DRUGS (ZOLPIDEM, ZALEPLON, AND ZOPICLONE)

Introduction: They are imidazopyridine derivative sedative and hypnotic which facilitate GABAergic transmission.
- Zopiclone
- Zolpidem-S enantiomer
- Zaleplon

Pharmacodynamics: Interacts with central nervous system (CNS) GABA benzodiazepine-chloride ionophore receptor complex.

Action is mediated by binding to BZD site of alpha 1 subunit containing GABA-A receptors increasing the frequency of chloride channel opening resulting in inhibition of neuronal excitation.

Pharmacokinetics:
- *Zolpidem*:
  - Bioavailability is 70% and peak plasma concentration attained in 1.5 hours.
  - Food decreased area under curve by 15%
  - Metabolized by CYP3A4
  - Half-life is 2.5–3 hours
  - Excreted principally in the urine
- *Zopiclone*:
  - T_{max} is 1 hour (fast acting)
  - High fat meal decreases peak plasma concentration by 21%
  - Metabolized by oxidation and demethylation CYP3A4 and CYP2E1
  - Half-life is 6 hours
  - Excreted in urine

- *Zaleplon*:
  - T_{max} is 1 hour (fast acting) and oral bioavailability is 30%
  - High fat meal decreases peak plasma concentration by 35%
  - Metabolized by aldehyde oxidase and lesser extent by CYP3A4
  - Half-life is 1 hour (short acting)
  - Excreted in urine

Uses (all three drugs):
- Short-term management of insomnia
- Mainly for sleep initiation
- Does not substantially increase total sleep time or increase number of awakening

Dose:
- *Zolpidem*: Oral (conventional and extended release) and sublingual 5–10 mg
  - Extended release:
    - Woman—6.25 mg
    - Men—6.25 or 12.5 mg
  - Sublingual-middle of night awakening:
    - Woman—1.75 mg
    - Men—3.5 mg
- *Zaleplon*:
  - Adults <65 years of age—10 mg initially
  - Maximum dose—20 mg
- *Eszopiclone*: 1 mg, may increase to 2–3 mg if clinically indicated, maximum 3 mg

Adverse effects:
- Common—drowsiness, dizziness, and diarrhea
- Complex sleep behaviors (parasomnias)
- Hypersensitivity
- Psychomotor impairment on the following day

Use in special population:
- *Pregnancy*: No association with major birth defects with zolpidem. Insufficient evidence for other drugs. May cross respiratory depression and sedation in neonates.
- Secreted in to breast milk
- Discontinue breast milk during treatment and after 2 hours
- Not recommended in pediatric patients
- Reduce dose in mild/moderate hepatic impairment
- Avoid in severe hepatic impairment, may precipitate encephalopathy
- No dose adjustment in renal failure

ZILUCOPLAN

Introduction: Small 15-amino acid macrocyclic peptide and inhibitor of complement C5.

Pharmacodynamics: Binds to complement protein C5 and inhibits its cleavage to C5a and C5b preventing the generation of C5b-9. Precise mechanism is unknown but it presumed to be involved reduction of C5b-9 deposition at neuromuscular junction.

Pharmacokinetics: Subcutaneous (SC) preparation. Half-life is 172 hours. Peak plasma time is 3–6 hours. Steady state through concentration reaches by 4–12 weeks. Metabolism is expected to be degraded into peptides and amino acids via catabolic pathway.

Uses: Indicated for generalized myasthenia gravis in adults who are acetylcholine receptor (AChR) antibody positive.

Dose: Dosage based on actual body weight:
- <56 kg: 16.6 mg SC QD
- 56 to <77 kg: 23 mg SC QD
- >77 kg: 32.4 mg SC QD

Adverse effects: Injection site reaction (29%), upper respiratory tract infection (URTI) (14%), diarrhea (11%), and less common are URTI, nausea, increased lipase, and amylase. Black box warning of increased risk of meningococcal infections (vaccinate 2 weeks before).

Use in special population: No data available for safety in pregnancy and lactation. No dosage adjustment needed in renal and hepatic impairment.

ZINC ACETATE

Introduction: Zinc acetate received approval by the United States Food and Drug Administration (US FDA) in 1997 for Wilson's disease. In other parts of the world, zinc sulfate is used and is equally effective.

Pharmacodynamics: Zinc acts by inhibiting the copper uptake from the gastrointestinal mucosa. Zinc induces enterocyte metallothionein, a cysteine-rich protein that has greater affinity for copper than for zinc thereby inhibiting copper entry into the portal circulation.

Pharmacokinetics: Half-life is 11 days following cessation of therapy. Excretion is in feces. Absorption PH dependent (enhanced at PH <3): Impaired by food.

Uses: As a first-line or second-line drug (along with other chelating agents) for Wilson's disease.

Dose: 50 mg PO three times daily in normal adults and during pregnancy 25 mg PO thrice daily and increase if there is inadequate response. It should be taken 30 minutes before or 2 hours after the meal. Efficacy of zinc acetate in treatment of Wilson's disease can be assessed by a goal of 24 urine copper values of <125 µg/day.

Adverse effects: The most common side effect of zinc treatment is gastric irritation, nausea, and vomiting. Rare side effects are pancreatitis (elevated lipase and amylase). Copper deficiency leading to anemia can occur in chronic use.

Use in special population: Studies in pregnant women showed no potential fetal harm and can be used. In lactating women it appears in breast milk and causes copper deficiency in babies and so should avoid breastfeeding. No data available for dose adjustment in renal and hepatic impairment perhaps it improve the hepatic and renal functions.

ZONISAMIDE

Introduction: Zonisamide is a sulfonamide antiepileptic drug that is a 1,2-benzisoxazole derivative.

Pharmacodynamics: Zonisamide acts through the blockade of voltage-dependent sodium and T-type calcium channels. It possibly also inhibits glutamate release. It is a weak carbonic anhydrase inhibitor, although this action is not responsible for its antiepileptic activity.

Pharmacokinetics: Half-life is 63 hours (plasma) and 105 hours [red blood cell (RBC)]. Peak plasma time is 2–6 hours. Metabolism is by CYP3A4. Excretion is in urine and feces. Bioavailability is high, but because of the lack of availability of a parenteral product, absolute bioavailability in humans is unknown.

Uses: It was FDA approved in the United States in 2000 for use as adjunctive therapy to treat partial seizures in adults. Small clinical studies have indicated that zonisamide is effective for other types of epilepsy and epilepsy syndromes such as infantile spasms, progressive myoclonus epilepsy, Lennox–Gastaut syndrome, simple partial seizures, complex partial seizures, and myoclonic seizures.

Dose: Initial 100 mg PO QD and can increase up to 200 mg/day after 2 weeks and may increase further by 100 mg/day after minimum of 2 weeks between adjustments. Not exceed 600 mg/day.

Adverse effects: Dizziness, somnolence, anorexia, ataxia, fatigue, abnormal thinking, and confusion are common side effects of zonisamide use.

Use in special population: Zonisamide is a pregnancy category C drug. Women of childbearing age should use effective birth control when taking zonisamide as it rapidly crosses the placenta. Risks and benefits must be weighed when using zonisamide during pregnancy. It appears in breast milk at similar levels to maternal plasma concentrations. Caution is advised, with slow titration and frequent monitoring in these patients. Use is not recommended for severe renal impairment (creatinine clearance < 20 mL/minute).

SECTION 2

Disease-based Catalogue of Drugs

Introduction

The second section provides a disease- or condition-based categorization of the drugs with appropriate classifications where necessary. Broad groups of neurological diseases have been arranged alphabetically with subsections of diseases under each category. This section provides a bird's eye view of drugs appropriate to each of the conditions. It also provides classification of drugs according to their use (e.g., acute vs. long-term/prophylaxis) or their mode of action where applicable.

Section Outline

- Autoimmune encephalitis
- Central and peripheral demyelinating disorders
- Dementia
- Epilepsy
- Headache and other craniofacial pain
- Nerve and muscle diseases
- Neurometabolic disorders
- Neuromuscular junction disorder
- Neuropathic pain
- Parkinson's disease
- Sleep disorders
- Stroke
- Symptomatic treatment

AUTOIMMUNE ENCEPHALITIS

- *First-line immunotherapies*:
  - Intravenous (IV) methylprednisolone pulse therapy
  - IV immunoglobulin
  - Plasma exchange
- *Second-line immunotherapies*:
  - Cyclophosphamide
  - Rituximab (particularly in NMDAR encephalitis)
- *Third-line immunotherapies (refractory NMDAR encephalitis and seronegative cases)*:
  - Bortezomib
  - Tocilizumab

CENTRAL AND PERIPHERAL DEMYELINATING DISORDERS

Multiple Sclerosis

- *Acute attack*:
  - IV methylprednisolone
  - Intravenous immunoglobulin (IVIg)
- *Disease-modifying agents*:
  - Injectable:
    - Interferon beta-1a and 1b (preferred in pregnancy)
    - Glatiramer acetate
  - Monoclonal antibodies (injectable):
    - Natalizumab
    - Alemtuzumab
    - Ocrelizumab [for primary progressive multiple sclerosis (PPMS)]
  - Oral:
    - Fingolimod
    - Ozanimod

- Siponimod
- Cladribine
- Teriflunomide
- Dimethyl fumarate
- Mitoxantrone
- Azathioprine

Neuromyelitis Optica Spectrum Disorders

- *Acute attack*:
  - IV methylprednisolone
  - IVIg
  - Plasma exchange
- *Immunosuppression to prevent relapses*:
  - Azathioprine
- *Monoclonal antibodies*:
  - Inebilizumab
  - Rituximab
  - Satralizumab
  - Eculizumab

Acute Disseminated Encephalomyelitis

- *Acute attack*:
  - IV methylprednisolone
  - IVIg
  - Plasma exchange

Myelin Oligodendrocyte Glycoprotein Antibody Disease

- *Acute attack*:
  - IV methylprednisolone
  - IVIg
  - Plasma exchange
- *Relapse prevention*:
  - Azathioprine
  - Rituximab

Peripheral Demyelinating Diseases

- *Acute inflammatory demyelinating polyneuropathy (AIDP)*:
  - IVIg
  - Plasma exchange
- *Chronic inflammatory demyelinating polyneuropathy (CIDP)*:
  - Rituximab
  - Corticosteroids

- Cyclophosphamide
- Cyclosporine and mycophenolate mofetil
- *Multifocal motor neuropathy (MMN)*:
  - IVIg

DEMENTIA

- *Drugs to improve memory*:
  - Cholinesterase inhibitors:
    - Donepezil
    - Rivastigmine
    - Galantamine
  - NMDAR antagonist:
    - Memantine
  - Monoclonal antibody:
    - Aducanumab
- *Drugs for behavioral symptoms*:
  - Antipsychotics:
    - Aripiprazole
    - Clozapine
    - Haloperidol
    - Olanzapine
    - Quetiapine
    - Risperidone
  - Antidepressants:
    - Escitalopram
    - Fluoxetine
    - Paroxetine
    - Sertraline
    - Venlafaxine
  - Mood stabilizers:
    - Valproate
    - Lamotrigine

EPILEPSY

- *Generalized*:
  - Valproic acid
  - Lamotrigine
  - Levetiracetam
  - Clonazepam
  - Ethosuximide
- *Focal*:
  - Acetazolamide
  - Brivaracetam
  - Carbamazepine
  - Clobazam

- Eslicarbazepine
- Ezogabine
- Felbamate
- Gabapentin
- Lacosamide
- Lamotrigine
- Oxcarbazepine
- Perampanel
- Phenobarbitone
- Phenytoin
- Pregabalin
- Rufinamide
- Topiramate
- Vigabatrin
- Zonisamide
- *Status epilepticus*:
    - Lorazepam
    - Midazolam
    - Diazepam
    - Fosphenytoin
    - Valproate
    - Levetiracetam
- *Refractory status epilepticus*:
    - Propofol
    - Ketamine
    - Immunoglobulin
- *Super refractory status epilepticus*:
    - Thiopentone

HEADACHE AND OTHER CRANIOFACIAL PAIN

Migraine

- *Acute attack*:
    - Nonsteroidal anti-inflammatory drug (NSAID)
        - Naproxen
        - Ketorolac
        - Aspirin
    - 5-HT agents:
        - Dihydroergotamine
        - Triptans
        - Almotriptan
        - Eletriptan
        - Frovatriptan
        - Naratriptan
        - Rizatriptan
        - Sumatriptan
        - Zolmitriptan

- Gepants [calcitonin gene-related peptide (CGRP) blocker]:
  - Atogepant
  - Rimegepant
  - Ubrogepant
  - Zavegepant
- Ditans: Lasmiditan

Prophylactic Therapy

Commonly used agents:
- Amitriptyline
- Nortriptyline
- Topiramate
- Valproic acid
- Gabapentin
- Propranolol
- Verapamil
- Magnesium
- Flunarizine
- *Gepants*:
  - Atogepant
  - Rimegepant

Monoclonal antibodies:
- *CGRP blockers*:
  - Erenumab
  - Eptinezumab
  - Galcanezumab
  - Fremanezumab

Status Migrainosus

- Dihydroergotamine
- Ketorolac
- IV valproic acid
- Dexamethasone
- Prochlorperazine
- IV magnesium

Trigeminal Autonomic Cephalalgia

- *Cluster headache*:
  - Acute
  - Triptans
  - 100% nasal oxygen (>12 L)
- *Transitional prophylaxis*:
  - Methylprednisolone/prednisolone
  - Verapamil

- *Paroxysmal hemicrania*:
  - Indomethacin
  - Sumatriptan
- *Hemicrania continua*:
  - Indomethacin
- Short-lasting unilateral neuralgiform headache attacks with conjunctival injection and tearing (SUNCT)/short-lasting unilateral neuralgiform headache attacks with cranial autonomic symptoms (SUNA):
  - Lamotrigine
  - Rescue-IV lignocaine
  - IV phenytoin

NERVE AND MUSCLE DISEASES

Nerve and Muscle Disorders

Muscle Disease

- *Duchenne muscular dystrophy*:
  - Ataluren
  - Casimersen
  - Deflazacort
  - Delandistrogene moxeparvovec
  - Eteplirsen
  - Givinostat
  - Golodirsen
- *Inflammatory myopathies*:
  - Methylprednisolone
  - IVIg
  - Methotrexate
  - Azathioprine
  - Cyclophosphamide
  - Cyclosporine
  - Tacrolimus
  - Rituximab
  - Tocilizumab
  - Mycophenolate mofetil

Myotonic Disorders

- Phenytoin
- Mexiletine

Mitochondrial Myopathies

- Coenzyme Q10

Channelopathies

- Acetazolamide

Motor Neuron Disease

Amyotrophic Lateral Sclerosis
- Riluzole
- Edaravone
- Tofersen

Spinomuscular Atrophy
- Risdiplam
- Nusinersen
- Onasemnogene abeparvovec

Motor Neuron Disease Variants
- *Brown-Vialetto-Van Laere*: Riboflavin
- *Fazio-Londe syndrome*: Riboflavin.

Diseases of Peripheral Nerves

Vasculitic Neuropathy
- *Induction*:
    - IV methylprednisolone
    - Cyclophosphamide
    - Rituximab
- *Maintenance*:
    - Methylprednisolone/prednisolone
    - Azathioprine
    - Mycophenolate mofetil
    - Methotrexate
- *Neuropathies due to deficiency*:
    - Ataxia with vitamin E deficiency—alpha tocopherol
    - Subacute combined degeneration—methylcobalamin
    - Dry beriberi—thiamine
    - Pyridoxine deficiency—pyridoxine

NEUROMETABOLIC DISORDERS

Neurometabolic

- *Wilson's disease*:
    - Chelation:
        - D-penicillamine
        - Trientine
    - Maintenance:
        - Ammonium tetrathiomolybdate
        - Zinc acetate
- *Porphyria*: Hematin
- *Pompe's disease*: Alglucosidase alfa

- *Carnitine deficiency*: L-carnitine
- *Cerebral folate deficiency*: Folic acid
- *Pyridoxine-dependent epilepsy*: Pyridoxine
- *Tyrosine hydroxylase deficiency*: Levodopa/carbidopa, selegiline, and rasagiline

NEUROMUSCULAR JUNCTION DISORDER

Myasthenia Gravis

- *Myasthenic crisis*:
  - IVIg
- *Maintenance therapy*:
  - Pyridostigmine
  - Neostigmine
  - Deflazacort
  - Methylprednisolone/prednisolone
  - Methotrexate
  - Mycophenolate mofetil
  - Azathioprine
  - Cyclophosphamide
  - Rituximab
  - Ravulizumab
  - Eculizumab
  - Rozanolixizumab
  - Efgartigimod
  - Tacrolimus
  - Cyclosporine

Lambert–Eaton Myasthenic Syndrome

- *Mild to moderate*:
  - Amifampridine
  - Pyridostigmine
- *Severe*:
  - Prednisolone
  - Azathioprine
  - IVIg

Congenital Myasthenic Syndromes

- *Most types*:
  - Pyridostigmine
  - Amifampridine
- *Slow channel*:
  - Fluoxetine
  - Quinidine
- *DOK7, agrin, and musk mutation*: Albuterol

NEUROPATHIC PAIN

- *Opioids*:
  - Tramadol
  - Tapentadol
- *Tricyclic antidepressants*:
  - Amitriptyline
  - Nortriptyline
  - Clomipramine
  - Desipramine
  - Dosulepin
  - Doxepin
  - Imipramine
- *Serotonin–norepinephrine reuptake inhibitor (SNRI)*:
  - Duloxetine
  - Venlafaxine
- *Anticonvulsants*:
  - Gabapentin
  - Pregabalin
  - Carbamazepine
  - Eslicarbazepine
  - Oxcarbazepine
  - Lamotrigine
  - Valproic acid
  - Topiramate
- *Topical*:
  - Lidocaine
  - Capsaicin
- *Fibromyalgia*:
  - Pregabalin
  - Duloxetine
  - Milnacipran
  - Amitriptyline
  - Nortriptyline

PARKINSON'S DISEASE

- *Anticholinergics*:
  - Benztropine
  - Trihexyphenidyl
  - Procyclidine
- *Dopamine precursors*:
  - Levodopa + carbidopa
  - Levodopa + benserazide
- *Dopamine agonists*:
  - Pramipexole
  - Cabergoline
  - Ropinirole
  - Rotigotine

- *COMT inhibitors*:
  - Entacapone
  - Tolcapone
  - Opicapone
- *MAO inhibitors*:
  - Rasagiline
  - Selegiline
  - Safinamide
- *Adenosine antagonist*: Istradefylline
- *Rescue therapy*: Apomorphine
- *Miscellaneous*: Amantadine

SLEEP DISORDERS

Wakefulness Promoting Agents

- Modafinil
- Armodafinil
- Pitolisant

Cataplexy

- Imipramine
- Sodium oxybate

Sleep Promoting Agents

- *Circadian rhythm disorders*: Melatonin
- *Sedatives*:
  - Benzodiazepines
  - Temazepam
  - Alprazolam
  - Clonazepam
  - Etizolam
  - Lemborexant
  - Suvorexant
  - Nonbenzodiazepine sedatives-Z drugs

STROKE

- *Reperfusion*:
  - Alteplase
  - Tenecteplase
- *Secondary prevention*:
  - Anticoagulants:
    - Oral:
      - Acenocoumarol
      - Apixaban
      - Rivaroxaban
      - Warfarin

- Injectable:
  - Heparin
  - Enoxaparin [low-molecular-weight heparin (LMWH)]
  - Fondaparinux
- Antiplatelet agents:
  - Aspirin
  - Clopidogrel
  - Cilostazol
  - Dipyridamole
  - Prasugrel
  - Ticagrelor
- Lipid-lowering agent:
  - Atorvastatin
  - Rosuvastatin
- *Neuroprotective*:
  - Citicoline
  - Edaravone
  - Sovateltide
  - Piracetam
- *Vasospasm prevention*: Nimodipine
- *Miscellaneous*: Nicergoline

SYMPTOMATIC TREATMENT

- *Chorea*:
  - Tetrabenazine
  - Valbenazine
  - Sodium valproate (rheumatic chorea)
  - Clonazepam
  - Diazepam
  - Haloperidol
- *Dystonia*:
  - Baclofen
  - Botulinum toxin
  - Trihexyphenidyl
  - Benztropine
  - Diazepam
  - Clonazepam
- *Tremor*:
  - Propranolol
  - Primidone
  - Clonazepam
  - Trihexyphenidyl
  - Benztropine
  - Procyclidine
  - Topiramate
- *Vertigo*:
  - Cinnarizine

- Meclizine
- Dimenhydrinate
- Betahistine
- Prochlorperazine
- Promethazine
- *Spasticity*:
    - Baclofen
    - Botulinum toxin
    - Tizanidine
    - Diazepam
- *Intractable hiccough*:
    - Chlorpromazine
    - Gabapentin
    - Baclofen
    - Ondansetron
- *Ataxia*:
    - Vitamin E
    - Riluzole
    - Amantadine
    - Dalfampridine
- *Overactive bladder*:
    - Mirabegron
    - Trospium
    - Darifenacin
    - Solifenacin
    - Tolterodine
    - Fesoterodine
    - Oxybutynin
- *Hypoactive bladder*: Bethanechol
- *Nocturnal enuresis*: Imipramine
- *Stress incontinence*: Duloxetine
- *Cerebral edema*:
    - Mannitol
    - Hypertonic saline
    - Dexamethasone
- *Orthostatic hypotension*:
    - Droxidopa
    - Fludrocortisone
    - Midodrine
- *Nystagmus*:
    - Gabapentin
    - Carbamazepine
- *Pseudobulbar affect*: Quinidine + dextromethorphan
- *Premature ejaculation*:
    - Paroxetine
    - Fluoxetine
    - Venlafaxine